365 Days of Aromatherapy Recipes

By: Coral James

365 Days of Aromatherapy Recipes

Table of Contents

Anti-Stress Aromatic Massage Oil
Sleep Inducing Aromatic Massage Oil

February

Aphrodisiac Massage Oil Blend
Sore Muscle Massage Oil Blend
Never Be Lonesome Diffuser Blend
Make Me Smile Diffuser Blend
Scented Hair Aromatic Blend
Hold Me Close Perfume Blend
Confidence Diffuser Blend
Make Him/Her Yours Diffuser Blend
Aromatic Bath Blend
Aromatic "Kiss Me" Mouthwash
Men's Sexy Cologne Blend
Aromatic Love Dust
Sensual Diffuser Blend
Romantic Dinner Diffuser Blend
Sensual Diffuser Blend
In The Mood Massage Oil
Romance Me Massage Oil
Let's Make Love Body Lotion
Romantic Encounter Body Lotion
Aphrodisiac Bath Soak
Sweetheart Diffuser Blend
Lover's Diffuser Blend
Exotic Evening Diffuser Blend
Perfect Passion Diffuser Blend
Love Is All Around Us Diffuser Blend
Lover's Desire Diffuser Blend
Sweetly Romantic Diffuser Blend
Hearts On Fire Diffuser Blend
Ring Around the Rosy Diffuser Blend

March

Immune Booster Diffuser Blend
Germs Be Gone Diffuser Blend

Feel Healthy Diffuser Blend
Say No to The Spring Sniffles Diffuser Blend
Fill My Home with Health Diffuser Blend
Say Goodbye to That Stubborn Headache Diffuser Blend
Aromatic Room Surface Spray Cleanser
Aromatic Lemon-Mint Cleaner
Aromatic Toilet Bowl Cleaner
Aromatic Glass Cleaner
Seasonal Discomfort Diffuser Blend
Common Cold Helper Diffuser Blend
Breathe Easy Diffuser Blend
Spring Breeze Diffuser Blend
Spring Man Cave Diffuser Blend
Aromatic Daily Shower Stall Spray
Aromatherapy St. Patty's Day Blend
Spring Bath Blend
Floral Bath Aromatic Blend
Aromatic Oven Cleaner
Aromatic Foaming Spring Hand Soap
Spring Love Potion Massage Oil
Spring Hand Massage Oil
Spring Head Massage Oil
Spring Nighttime Foot Massage Oil
Love My Face Spring Massage Oil
Get Those Legs Going Massage Oil
I Love Spring Diffuser Oil Blend
Candy Shop Diffuser Oil Blend
Spring Forest Diffuser Oil Blend
So Fresh and So Clean Diffuser Oil Blend

April

Stay Focused Diffuser Oil Blend
Citrus Overload Diffuser Oil Blend
Odor Buster Diffuser Oil Blend
Pretty Flowers Diffuser Oil Blend
Calm Down Diffuser Oil Blend
Grounding Diffuser Oil Blend
Slow Down Diffuser Oil Blend
Set My Emotions Straight Diffuser Oil Blend

May

June

Summer Rain Diffuser Blend
Yoga Diffuser Blend
Mountain Breeze Diffuser Blend
Peaceful Little One Diffuser Blend
Summer Workout Diffuser Blend
Summer Snuggles Diffuser Blend
Summer Stink Buster Diffuser Blend
Moonlit Path Diffuser Blend
Summer Friendship Diffuser Blend

July

Bugs Be Gone Diffuser Blend
Summer Slumber Diffuser Blend
Hanging Out at Home Diffuser Blend
Relax On My Lap Diffuser Blend
Sweet Summer Daydreams Diffuser Blend
Naptime Diffuser Blend
Sleepy Smiles Diffuser Blend
Happy Dreams Diffuser Blend
Insect Blaster Aromatic Spray
Aerobics Time Diffuser Blend
Staycation Diffuser Blend
Exotic Vacation Diffuser Blend
Summer Sweetie Diffuser Blend
Sunshiny Day Diffuser Blend
Tahitian Vacation Diffuser Blend
Alpine Dreams On A Summer Day Diffuser Blend
Jet Lag Morning Mist
Jet Lag Evening Mist
Bugs Be Gone Diffuser Blend
You're getting On My Nerves Diffuser Blend
Island Vacation Diffuser Blend
Get Herbal Summer Diffuser Blend
Aromatic Car Diffuser Blend
Get Up and Get Stuff Done Diffuser Blend
Mojito Diffuser Blend
I Am Woman Summer Blend Diffuser Blend
Summer Treehouse Diffuser Blend
Cali Coast Diffuser Blend

August

September

Wake Up for School Diffuser Blend
Remember What You Learned Diffuser Blend
Protect My Health, Mom Diffuser Blend
Stay Calm During That Test Diffuser Blend
Happy Yummy Diffuser Blend
Aromatic Acne Buster Face Wash
Aromatic Solution for A Stinky Backpack
Aromatic Armpit Odor Buster
Dorm Room Deodorizer
Stop Stinking Up My Space, Puppy Dog
College Kid Car Deodorizer
Freshen Up Furniture Spray
Frat Boy Freezer Freshener
Instant Classroom Calmer Diffuser Blend
Calming Aromatherapy Rice Box
Natural Classroom Air Freshener
Aromatic Cloud Dough
Aromatic Plant Therapy
Study Time Diffuser Blend
Concentration Diffuser Blend
Wrap Your Mind Around Your Work Diffuser Blend
I Want to Learn Diffuser Blend
Reading Nook Diffuser Blend
School is Cool Diffuser Blend
Before School Diffuser Blend
Take to School Aromatic Roller Blend
Go Away College Cootie Diffuser Blend
Soothing Sugar Scrub Blend
Grumpy Kids Be Gone Diffuser Blend
Bake My Bad Mood Away (Cinnamon Rolls)

October

Pumpkin Pie Diffuser Blend
Autumn Spice Diffuser Blend
Spiced Chai Diffuser Blend
Walk in the Autumn Woods Diffuser Blend
Fall Family Hike Diffuser Blend
Falling Leaves Diffuser Blend
Spicy Citrus Diffuser Blend

Fall Sniffle Snuffer Diffuser Blend
Autumn Air Diffuser Blend
Spicy Cinnamon Diffuser Blend
Fall Wreath Diffuser Blend
Aromatic Autumn Perfume Blend
Fall Essential Oil Diffuser Necklace
Pumpkin Spice Sugar Scrub
Aromatic Autumn Potpourri Blend
Fall Pot Simmer
Autumn Room Mist
Woodsy, Fall Room Mist
Vanilla Passion Diffuser Blend
Pumpkin Pie Soap
Aromatic Fall Scented Sachet
Apple Pie Diffuser Blend
Fall Retreat Diffuser Blend
Crisp, Fall Day Cuddles Diffuser Blend
Spiced Cider Diffuser Blend
Fall Flannel Shirt Diffuser Blend
Snickerdoodle Diffuser Blend
Mulled Cider Diffuser Blend
Sweater Weather Diffuser Blend
Candy Bowl Diffuser Blend
Trick or Treat Diffuser Blend

November

Fresh Stuffing Diffuser Blend
Mother's November Brew Diffuser Blend
Be Thankful, Dear Child Diffuser Blend
Sweet, November Nights Diffuser Blend
Pumpkin Bread Diffuser Blend
Spiced Tea Diffuser Blend
Harvest Time Diffuser Blend
Turkey Dinner Diffuser Blend
Run into The Woods Diffuser Blend
Fresh, Baked Pumpkin Pie Recipe
November Day Diffuser Blend
Peaceful, November Night's Sleep Diffuser Blend
Vivid Dreams Diffuser Blend

No More Grouchies Diffuser Blend
Autumn Zing Diffuser Blend
Thanksgiving Dinner Diffuser Blend
Oatmeal Cookie Diffuser Blend
Give Thanks Diffuser Blend
Orange Pomander Diffuser Blend
Thankful Heart Diffuser Blend
Orange Glow Diffuser Blend
Fresh, Fall Home Diffuser Blend
Here Comes the Harvest Sun Diffuser Blend
Northern Lights Diffuser Blend
Under the Blankets Diffuser Blend
Pumpkin Latte Diffuser Blend
Fall Festival Diffuser Blend
Pumpkin Spice Pot Simmer
Fall Travels Diffuser Blend
Cinnamon Creamsicle Diffuser Blend

December

Christmas Tree Farm Diffuser Blend
Christmas Candy Diffuser Blend
Peaceful Holiday Farm Diffuser Blend
Spicy Christmas Candy Diffuser Blend
Winter Christmas Tree Diffuser Blend
Winter Wonder Diffuser Blend
Solstice Celebration Diffuser Blend
Winter Happiness Diffuser Blend
Orange Cream Diffuser Blend
Candy Cane Diffuser Blend
Black Licorice Diffuser Blend
Gingerbread Man Diffuser Blend
Santa's Workshop Diffuser Blend
Candy Cane Forest Diffuser Blend
Sea of Swirly Twirly Gumdrops Diffuser Blend
Christmas Coffee Diffuser Blend
Snow Angels Diffuser Blend
Christmas Cheer Diffuser Blend
Christmas Cookie Recipe
Peppermint Surprise Diffuser Blend

Conclusion

<u>Introduction</u>

Hello! Welcome to learning about the many wonders of aromatherapy and what it can do for your life. This book has been designed to give you easy-to-create aromatherapy recipes for each day of the year. You'll be amazed at the power of essential oils and how they can fill your life and home with intriguing scents that alleviate the stresses of life and brighten your mood. There are aromatherapy combinations for every season of life and this book is going to help you experiment with 365 different combinations. From aromatic massage oils to specific diffuser blends, you'll find it all in 365 Days of Aromatherapy Recipes.

<u>What is Aromatherapy?</u>

Did you know that aromatherapy is also known as essential oil therapy? When we use aromatherapy, we are utilizing the art and science of naturally extracted aromatic essences from plants to bring balance, harmony, and good health to our bodies, minds, and spirits.

"It was the French perfumer and chemist, Rene-Maurice Gattefosse, who coined the term "aromatherapie" in 1937 with his publication of a book by that name. His book "Gattefosse's Aromatherapy" contains early clinical findings for utilizing essential oils for a range of physiological ailments. It seems vital to understand what Gattefosse's intention for coining the word was, as he clearly meant to distinguish the medicinal application of essential oils from their perfumery applications."

"Aromatherapy is... the skilled and controlled use of essential oils for physical and emotional health and well-being." Valerie Cooksley

"Aromatherapy is a caring, hands-on therapy which seeks to induce relaxation, to increase energy, to reduce the effects of stress and to restore lost balance to mind, body and soul." Robert Tisserand

"Aromatherapy can be defined as the controlled use of essential oils to maintain and promote physical, psychological, and spiritual wellbeing." Gabriel Mojay

"Aromatherapy can be defined as the art and science of utilizing naturally extracted aromatic es-

sences from plants to balance, harmonize and promote the health of body, mind and spirit. It is an art and science which seeks to explore the physiological, psychological and spiritual realm of the individual's response to aromatic extracts as well as to observe and enhance the individual's innate healing process. As a holistic practice, Aromatherapy is both a preventative approach as well as an active method to employ during acute and chronic stages of illness or 'dis'-ease."

"It is a natural, non-invasive modality designed to affect the whole person not just the symptom or disease and to assist the body's natural ability to balance, regulate, heal and maintain itself by the correct use of essential oils." Jade Shutes

Source: https://www.naha.org/explore-aromatherapy/about-aromatherapy/what-is-aromatherapy/

<u>Types of Aromatherapy</u>

"There are three main uses of aromatherapy. They are categorized keeping in mind that not all aromatic oils should be applied on the skin directly. While certain oils can only be beneficial if used in the form of inhalation, others help when applied topically."

1. Aromatherapy using only the Fragrance or Sense of Smell or Olfaction:

In this method of aromatherapy, essential oils are perceived through the sense of smell to give a therapeutic benefit. This is done by a direct or indirect inhalation or aerial diffusion of essential oils. Olfactory Aromatherapy is beneficial because the brain is conditioned from memory for various kinds of odors. This is made use of to synchronize and regulate the natural forces of the body to establish an innate balance and peace.

2. Cosmetic Aromatherapy

The essential oils used on the body as a moisturizer, cleanser, skin and hair care products come under this category. The cosmetic industry is currently utilizing the benefits of aromatherapy to revitalize and rejuvenate the body besides catering to the essential cleaning, toning, moisturizing and protective properties of essential oils for various skin and hair types.

3. Aromatherapy using Massage or Topical Application:

Essential oils can be absorbed through the skin by massage or topical application. This promotes a holistic healing of the whole body by traveling through the bloodstream and affecting various organs of the body. Some of these oils are also potent anti-viral, antifungal and antiseptic in nature. This, coupled with the sense of touch is a completely natural and safe way of detoxifying and making use of nature's bounty!

Thank you to Medindia for this very helpful list of types of aromatherapy and how they can be used to benefit the body, mind, and soul.

Source:
http://www.medindia.net/alternativemedicine/aromatherapy/aromatherapy-types.htm

January

Ah, the month of January is upon us and this means winter blues, dry skin, and brittle hair. However, it doesn't have to be this way! This chapter focuses on ways to take care of yourself during winter's harshest month, and getting a healthy dose of aromatherapy as you do. You'll find diffuser recipes, lotions, bath washes, shampoos, and much more that'll leave your body feeling great and your senses filled with an exhilaration only aromatherapy can provide.

January 1

Comforting Digestive Support Blend

Materials

- Cardamom Essential Oil – 10 drops

- Ginger Essential Oil – 10 drops

- Tarragon Essential Oil – 5 drops

Directions

Blend essential oils and shake well. Use this aromatherapy blend to encourage proper winter digestive health by adding to your diffuser, massaging directly onto your stomach (use a carrier oil), or adding 3 drops to your morning cup of tea mixed with a bit of milk.

January 2

Flu and Sinus Congestion Blend

Materials

- Niaouli Essential Oil – 6 tsp.

- Rosemary Essential Oil – 3 tsp.

- Pine Essential Oil – 3 tsp.

- Lavender Essential Oil – 2 tsp.

- Lemon Essential Oil – 2 tsp.

- Alcohol (90%) – 4 ½ cups

Directions

Mix all ingredients together. You may use this concoction as an inhalant by adding 3 tbsps. to 6 cups of boiling water. This blend can also be added to foot soaks and tub baths, a few drops at a time.

January 3

Woodsy Winter Welcome Diffuser Blend

Materials

- Pine Essential Oil – 3 drops

- Black Pepper Essential Oil – 2 drops

- Grapefruit Essential Oil – 5 drops

Directions

Add essential oils to your diffuser.

January 4

Winter Zing Diffuser Blend

Materials

- Frankincense Essential Oil – 5 drops

- Lemon Essential Oil – 5 drops

- Idaho Balsam Fir Essential Oil – 3 drops

Directions

Add essential oils to your diffuser.

January 5

Winter's Night Diffuser Blend

Materials

- Bergamot Essential Oil – 5 drops
- Northern Lights Black Spruce Essential Oil – 5 drops

Directions

Add essential oils to your diffuser.

January 6

Winter Royalty Diffuser Blend

Materials

- Royal Hawaiian Sandalwood Essential Oil – 5 drops
- Coriander Essential Oil – 5 drops

Directions

Add essential oils to your diffuser.

January 7

Warm Winter Blessing Diffuser Blend

Materials

- Cedar wood Essential Oil – 5 drops
- Cardamom Essential Oil – 4 drops

Directions

Add essential oils to your diffuser.

January 8

Fresh from the Bakery Blend

Materials

- Lemon Essential Oil – 5 drops
- Marjoram Essential Oil – 3 drops

Directions

Add essential oils to your diffuser.

January 9

Grandma's Winter Kitchen Diffuser Blend

Materials

- Tangerine Essential Oil – 5 drops
- Nutmeg Essential Oil – 3 drops

Directions

Add essential oils to your diffuser.

January 10

Grandpa's Winter Jacket Diffuser Blend

Materials

- Cinnamon Bark Essential Oil – 5 drops
- Lime Essential Oil – 3 drops

Directions

Add essential oils to your diffuser.

January 11

Warm Winter Dreams Diffuser Blend

Materials

- Orange Essential Oil – 5 drops

- Tarragon Essential Oil – 3 drops

Directions

Add essential oils to your diffuser.

January 12

Stay Well Winter Diffuser Blend

Materials

- Ginger Essential Oil – 2 drops

- Cinnamon Bark Essential Oil – 3 drops

- Grapefruit Essential Oil – 5 drops

Directions

Add essential oils to your diffuser.

January 13

Winter Aromatic Body Wash

Materials

- 3 tbsps. Liquid Castile Soap

- 3 tbsps. Raw Honey

- 1 tbsp. each of castor and olive oil

- Cinnamon Leaf Essential Oil – 10 drops

Directions

Mix all ingredients together in a glass mixing cup and carefully pour into a container that you can safely keep in the shower.

January 14

Skin Nourishing Winter Cleansing Oil

Materials

- 12 ounces' jojoba Oil

- 4 1/2 ounces' macadamia Oil

- 30 drops carrot seed Essential Oil

- 30 drops rose Essential Oil

Directions

Combine all ingredients and store in an airtight container. Apply to dry skin, twice daily or as your beauty treatment before bed. The scent aromatic scent of rose will help you sleep.

January 15

Beautifying Winter Body Butter

Materials

- 8 ounces' organic cocoa butter

- ½ cup sweet almond oil

- 1 ½ tsp. vanilla Essential Oil

Directions

Melt cocoa butter in a saucepan over gentle heat. Add sweet almond oil and continue heating until the liquid has just clarified. Remove from heat and stir in the essential oil. Allow to cool and store in an airtight container.

January 16

Simply Savvy Winter Aromatherapy Shaving Cream

Materials

- 2 tbsps. tamanu oil

- 2 tbsps. sweet almond oil

- 2 tbsps. cocoa butter or shea butter

- 1 ½ cups distilled water

- 1 tsp. baking soda

- 4 tbsps. Castile soap

- ½ cup aloe vera gel or honey

- 12 drops lavender Essential Oil

Directions

Heat the tamanu and sweet almond oils and butter in a double boiler over a low heat. Stir until the mixture is clear, then pour into a large bowl and let cool.

In another pan, heat the water. Then add the baking soda and castile soap, stirring until completely diluted. Add the aloe vera gel or honey to this solution and stir.

Pour the soap mixture into the bowl with the now-room-temperature oil mixture. Add essential oil. Blend everything very well with a hand mixer or blender. For best results, blend for two minutes, stop and then blend again for another two minutes.

Store the cream in an airtight container in a dark, cool location.

Source: https://www.auracacia.com/recipes/tamanu-lavender-shaving-cream

January 17

Aromatic Winter Foot Oil

Materials

- 1-ounce tamanu oil

- 4 drops tea tree essential oil

- 4 drops peppermint essential oil

- 4 drops sandalwood essential oil

Directions

Blend essential oils into tamanu oil and apply to feet at least twice a day to relieve dry skin. Breath the essential oils in deeply as you work them into your tired toes.

January 18

Aromatic Moisturizing Face Mist

Materials

- 2 ounces' neroli hydrosol or purified water

- 1-ounce vegetable glycerin

- 1-ounce aloe vera gel juice

- 48 drops coriander seed essential oil

Directions

Combine all ingredients in a 4-ounce spray mister bottle, cap, and shake. Always shake bottle before misting solution onto the face.

January 19

Energizing Winter Coffee Body Scrub

Materials

- 1 cup sweet almond oil
- ¼ cup cacao nibs, crushed into granules
- ¼ cup granulated sugar
- 1 tsp. coffee grounds
- 1 tsp. vanilla essential oil

Directions

Add the almond oil to a pan and place over low heat. Add the nibs to the oil and heat until their own oils have released and settled onto the bottom of the pan. Remove pan from heat and allow to cool. Add sugar, coffee grounds, and essential oil to the pan and stir until evenly combined. Store in an air tight container.

January 20

Aromatic Hand and Foot Dip

Materials

- ½ lb. beeswax or soy wax
- 2 ounces' sweet almond oil
- ½ cup dried rose petals, crushed
- 24 drops lavender essential oil

Directions

Melt wax in a double boiler or bowl set in simmering water. Make sure the wax vessel is large enough to dip a hand or foot into. While wax is melting, mix the lavender essential oil into the sweet almond oil in a separate container. Crumble the rose petals into the melting wax. Once wax is fully melted, remove from heat and let cool. Use a meat or candy thermometer to measure 120 degrees. Pour half of the lavender-scented sweet almond oil into the melted wax mixture and stir. Coat hands or feet with the remaining lavender-scented sweet almond oil. Once the melted wax mixture reaches 110 degrees dip your hands or feet into the mixture and remove to let a skin form. Repeat until several layers of warm wax form on your skin. Have someone help you to wrap your hands or feet in plastic wrap and a warm towel or blanket. After 20 minutes, unwrap and peel away the wax and discard.

Source: https://www.auracacia.com/recipes/nurturing-rose-and-calming-lavender-warm-wax-hand-and-foot-dip

January 21

Aromatic Dry Dog Shampoo

Materials

- ¼ cup baking soda

- 10 drops lavender essential oil

Directions

Add ingredients to a container and mix. Use a shaker lid to easily apply to dog's fur. Work the product in with your hands.

January 22

Beat the Winter Blues Diffuser Blend

Materials

- 1 drop Ylang Ylang essential oil
- 4 drops orange essential oil

Directions

Place blend into your diffuser.

January 23

You Haven't Got a Hold On Me Old Man Winter Diffuser Blend

Materials

- 3 drops grapefruit essential oil
- 2 drops cypress essential oil

Directions

Place blend into your diffuser.

January 24

Cast Your Cares Diffuser Blend

Materials

- 3 drops bergamot essential oil
- 2 drops clary sage essential oil

Directions

Place blend into your diffuser.

January 25

Sittin' Pretty Winter's Day Diffuser Blend

Materials

- 3 drops bergamot essential oil

- 1 drop neroli essential oil

- 1 drop Jasmine

Directions

Place blend into your diffuser.

January 26

Say Good Bye to Winter Stink Air Freshener

Materials

- 15 drops bergamot essential oil

- 15 drops spearmint essential oil

- 1.5 fl. ounces' distilled water

- 1.5 fl. ounces' high-proof alcohol

Directions

Add all ingredients to a 4-ounce spray bottle, cap, and shake. Spray around the home or office as necessary.

January 27

Winter Woes Be Gone Air Freshener

Materials

- 20 drops lime essential oil

- 14 drops bergamot essential oil

- 4 drops ylang ylang

- 2 drops rose

- 1.5 fl. ounces' distilled water

- 1.5 fl. ounces' high-proof alcohol

Directions

Add all ingredients to a 4-ounce spray bottle, cap, and shake. Spray around the home or office as necessary.

January 28

So Long Winter Sadness Air Freshener

Materials

- 15 drops clary sage essential oil

- 9 drops lemon essential oil

- 6 drops lavender essential oil

- 1.5 fl. ounces' distilled water

- 1.5 fl. ounces' high-proof alcohol

Directions

Add all ingredients to a 4-ounce spray bottle, cap, and shake. Spray around the home or office as necessary.

January 29

Winter Won't Be Here Forever Air Freshener

Materials

- 20 drops rosemary essential oil

- 8 drops grapefruit essential oil

- 4 drops peppermint essential oil

- 2 drops spearmint essential oil

- 1.5 fl. ounces' distilled water

- 1.5 fl. ounces' high-proof alcohol

Directions

Add all ingredients to a 4-ounce spray bottle, cap, and shake. Spray around the home or office as necessary.

January 30

Anti-Stress Aromatic Massage Oil

Materials

- 6 drops clary sage essential oil

- 2 drops lemon essential oil

- 3 drops lavender essential oil

- 1 fl. ounce carrier oil

Directions

Mix all oils and store in an airtight, glass container. Massage small amount into skin as needed.

January 31

Sleep Inducing Aromatic Massage Oil

Materials

- 10 drops Roman chamomile essential oil

- 1 fl. ounce carrier oil

Directions

Mix all oils and store in an airtight, glass container. Massage small amount into skin as needed.

February

February is the month of love so let's celebrate with a batch of aroma-therapy recipes that'll truly put you at the end of Cupid's arrow. From tantalizing massage oils that you and your lover can use to aromatic diffuser blends that set the mood of romance in your home, this chapter has it all.

February 1

Aphrodisiac Massage Oil Blend

Materials

- 8 drops sandalwood essential oil

- 2 drops Jasmine essential oil

Directions

Mix all oils and store in an airtight, glass container. Massage small amount into skin as needed.

February 2

Sore Muscle Massage Oil Blend

Materials

- 2 drops ginger essential oil

- 1 drop black pepper essential oil

- 4 drops peppermint essential oil

- 5 drops eucalyptus essential oil

Directions

Mix all oils and store in an airtight, glass container. Massage small amount into skin as needed.

February 3

Never Be Lonesome Diffuser Blend

Materials

- 1 drop rose essential oil

- 2 drops frankincense essential oil

- 2 drops bergamot

Directions

Add essential oils to your diffuser.

February 4

Make Me Smile Diffuser Blend

Materials

- 3 drops clary sage essential oil

- 2 drops bergamot essential oil

Directions

Add essential oils to your diffuser.

February 5

Scented Hair Aromatic Blend

Materials

- 1 drop rosemary, lavender, or sandalwood

- Bristle brush

Directions

Place one drop of essential oil to your favorite bristle brush and brush your hair.

February 6

Hold Me Close Perfume Blend

Materials

- 9 drops sandalwood EO

- 3 drops of either rose, jasmine, or neroli EO

- 1 tbsp. jojoba oil

Directions

Mix all ingredients together well and store in an airtight glass container, preferably dark colored. Dab a drop or two onto your pulse points.

February 7

Confidence Diffuser Blend

Materials

- 2 drops bay laurel

- 3 drops bergamot

Directions

Add essential oils to your diffuser. The perfect blend to diffuse before a big date!

February 8

Make Him/Her Yours Diffuser Blend

Materials

- 1 drop Jasmine

- 4 drops bergamot

Directions

Add essential oils to your diffuser. Diffuse this oil to seduce your lover.

February 9

Aromatic Bath Blend

Materials

- 2 fl. ounces' jojoba oil

- 20 drops lavender EO

Directions

Blend the oils together and store in a glass jar. Add a tablespoon or two to your bath water.

February 10

Aromatic "Kiss Me" Mouthwash

Materials

- 6 fl. ounces' water

- 1-2 fl. ounces' vodka

- 8 drops peppermint or spearmint EO

- 5 drops myrrh EO

Directions

Mix the water and vodka together in an 8-ounce bottle. Add the essential oils, shake well. Use as a mouth rinse after brushing teeth.

February 11

Men's Sexy Cologne Blend

Materials

- 2.5 fl. ounces' high proof vodka

- 1 fl. ounce distilled water

- 15 drops bergamot or mandarin EO

- 15 drops patchouli EO

- 5 drops bay laurel EO

- 3 drops black pepper or ginger EO

- 5 drops Oakmoss Absolute or 2-3 drops vetiver EO

- 1-2 drops neroli EO

Directions

Place the water and vodka in a 4-ounce glass bottle then add the oils. Cap the bottle and shake until evenly mixed. Allow the cologne to sit for several days, shaking 1-2 times per day before using.

February 12

Aromatic Love Dust

Materials

- 30 drops lavender EO

- 4 ounces' arrowroot powder

- Sifter container

Directions

Add the arrowroot powder to a mixing bowl followed by the essential oil. Mix with a fork to evenly distribute the oil throughout the powder. Transfer powder to a sifter bottle and use on your body.

February 13

Sensual Diffuser Blend

Materials

- 7 drops sandalwood

- 2 drops vanilla

- 1 drop ylang ylang

Directions

Add essential oils to your diffuser.

February 14

Romantic Dinner Diffuser Blend

Materials

- 2 drops each pf black pepper, grapefruit, and jasmine

Directions

Add essential oils to your diffuser.

February 15

Sensual Diffuser Blend

Materials

- 7 drops sandalwood
- 2 drops vanilla
- 1 drop ylang ylang

Directions

Add essential oils to your diffuser.

February 16

In The Mood Massage Oil

Materials

- 2 drops cedarwood
- 2 drops clary sage
- 1 drop orange
- 5 drops vanilla in jojoba oil
- 1-ounce carrier oil

Directions

Mix all oils together in a glass jar.

February 17

Romance Me Massage Oil

Materials

- 2 drops jasmine

- 2 drops orange

- 2 drops sandlewood

- 1 drop ylang ylang

- 1-ounce carrier oil

Directions

Mix all oils together in a glass jar.

February 18

Let's Make Love Body Lotion

Materials

- 2 drops rose

- 3 drops sandalwood

- 2 tbsps. unscented lotion

Directions

Combine oils with lotion and apply to face and body.

February 19

Romantic Encounter Body Lotion

Materials

- 2 drops ylang ylang

- 2 drops jasmine

- 2 drops bergamot

- 2 tbsps. unscented lotion

Directions

Combine oils with lotion and apply to face and body.

February 20

Aphrodisiac Bath Soak

Materials

- 4 drops jasmine

- 4 drops ginger

- 4 drops neroli

- 6 drops clary sage

- 1 drop black pepper

- 8 oz. milk

Directions

Combine oils in 8 ounces of milk and add to hot bath water.

February 21

Sweetheart Diffuser Blend

Materials

- 2 drops ylang ylang

- 8 drops sweet orange

- 2 drops lavender

Directions

Add oils to your diffuser.

February 22

Lover's Diffuser Blend

Materials

- 4 drops ylang ylang
- 2 drops mandarin
- 1 drop sandalwood
- 1 drop cedarwood

Directions

Add oils to your diffuser.

February 23

Exotic Evening Diffuser Blend

Materials

- 2 drops ylang ylang
- 3 drops sweet orange

Directions

Add oils to your diffuser.

February 24

Perfect Passion Diffuser Blend

Materials

- 5 drops geranium
- 6 drops jasmine

Directions

Add oils to your diffuser.

February 25

Love Is All Around Us Diffuser Blend

Materials

- 1 drop patchouli
- 3 drops jasmine
- 5 drops geranium

Directions

Add oils to your diffuser.

February 26

Lover's Desire Diffuser Blend

Materials

- 2 drops ylang ylang
- 2 drops chamomile

Directions

Add oils to your diffuser.

February 27

Sweetly Romantic Diffuser Blend

Materials

- 2 drops cedarwood

- 2 drops clary sage
- 7 drops vanilla
- 1 drops sweet orange

Directions

Add oils to your diffuser.

February 28

Hearts On Fire Diffuser Blend

Materials

- 6 drops tangerine
- 4 drops cinnamon bark
- 2 drops nutmeg

Directions

Add oils to your diffuser.

February 29

Ring Around the Rosy Diffuser Blend

Materials

- 1 drops geranium
- 15 drops rose

Directions

Add oils to your diffuser.

March

Finally, spring is creeping up on us! I don't know about you but I'm excited to say tell Old Man Winter to hit the road and hello to spring. The month of March will focus on immune boosting aromatherapy recipes and the start of our spring cleaning aromatic concoctions.

March 1

Immune Booster Diffuser Blend

Materials

- 2 drops rosemary
- 2 drops clove
- 2 drops eucalyptus
- 2 drops cinnamon
- 2 drops wild orange

Directions

Place all oils into your diffuser.

March 2

Germs Be Gone Diffuser Blend

Materials

- 2 drops lemon
- 2 drops oregano

Directions

Place all oils into your diffuser.

March 3

Feel Healthy Diffuser Blend

Materials

- 2 drops lemon

- 2 drops melaleuca

Directions

Place all oils into your diffuser.

March 4

Say No to The Spring Sniffles Diffuser Blend

Materials

- 1 drop rosemary

- 2 drops lemon

- 1 drop lime

- 2 drops peppermint

- 2 drops eucalyptus

- 1 drop clove

Directions

Place all oils into your diffuser.

March 5

Fill My Home with Health Diffuser Blend

Materials

- 2 drops rosemary

- 2 drops clove

- 2 drops eucalyptus

- 2 drops cinnamon

- 2 drops wild orange

Directions

Place all oils into your diffuser.

March 6

Say Goodbye to That Stubborn Headache Diffuser Blend

Materials

- 2 drops rosemary

- 2 drops marjoram

- 2 drops thyme

- 2 drops peppermint

- 2 drops lavender

Directions

Place all oils into your diffuser.

March 7

Aromatic Room Surface Spray Cleanser

Materials

- 25 drops ravensara

- 15 drops lavender

- 10 drops lemongrass

- 1 tsp. emulsifier

- 2 oz. non-toxic all-purpose cleaner (Try Shaklee)

Directions

Blend the essential oils together and add them to the emulsifier. Mix the solution to the all-purpose cleaner, cap, and shake well. Use to clean just about any surface.

March 8

Aromatic Lemon-Mint Cleaner

Materials

- 40 drops lemon

- 5 drops peppermint

- 1 tsp. emulsifier

- 2 oz. non-toxic all-purpose cleaner (Try Shaklee)

Directions

Blend the essential oils together and add them to the emulsifier. Mix the solution to the all-purpose cleaner, cap, and shake well. Use to clean just about any surface.

March 9

Aromatic Toilet Bowl Cleaner

Materials

- 50 drops lemon

- 1 cup baking soda

- 4 tbsps. white vinegar

Directions

Mix the essential oil with the baking soda and stir together with a fork. Store in an airtight glass jar. When ready to use, mix 2 tbsps. of baking soda mixture with 4 tbsps. of white vinegar in your toilet. Scrub with your toilet brush.

March 10

Aromatic Glass Cleaner

Materials

- 8 drops lime

- 1 ½ cup white vinegar

- ½ cup distilled water

Directions

Add all ingredients to a 16 oz. spray bottle, cap, and shake. Use on mirrors, windows, and basically any glass surface.

March 11

Seasonal Discomfort Diffuser Blend

Materials

- 3 drops lemon

- 3 drops lavender

- 3 drops peppermint

Directions

Add essential oils to your diffuser.

March 12

Common Cold Helper Diffuser Blend

Materials

- 5 drops rosemary
- 4 drops eucalyptus
- 4 drops peppermint
- 3 drops cypress
- 2 drops lemon

Directions

Add essential oils to your diffuser.

March 13

Breathe Easy Diffuser Blend

Materials

- 5 drops eucalyptus
- 4 drops peppermint

Directions

Add essential oils to your diffuser.

March 14

Spring Breeze Diffuser Blend

Materials

- 3 drops lemon

- 2 drops melaleuca

- 2 drops lime

- 2 drops white fir

- 2 drops cilantro

Directions

Add essential oils to your diffuser.

March 15

Spring Man Cave Diffuser Blend

Materials

- 3 drops bergamot

- 3 drops cypress

- 3 drops arborvitae

Directions

Add essential oils to your diffuser.

March 16

Aromatic Daily Shower Stall Spray

Materials

- 1 ½ cups water

- 1 cup white vinegar

- ½ cup rubbing alcohol

- 1 tsp. liquid dish soap

- 15 drops lemon

- 15 drops melaleuca

Directions

Add all ingredients to a spray bottle in the order in which they are listed, cap, shake. Use after each shower use.

March 17

Aromatherapy St. Patty's Day Blend

Materials

- 4 oz. distilled water

- Tiny, green crystal chips

- 4 oz. spray bottle

- 20 drops spearmint

- 10 drops vanilla

- 5 drops peppermint

Directions

Add the essential oils to the bottle followed by the water. Close the bottle and gentle swirl the water and oils. Reopen the bottle and add the crystal chips. Spray this lovely St. Patty's Day scent throughout your home.

March 18

Spring Bath Blend

Materials

- 1 drop jasmine

- 2 drops rose

- 10 drops bergamot

- ¼ cup carrier oil

Directions

Mix the essential oil with the carrier oil and pour under running bath water.

March 19

Floral Bath Aromatic Blend

Materials

- 2 drops lavender

- 1 drop German chamomile

- 2 drops ylang ylang

- 12 drops sweet orange

- 1/3 cup carrier oil

Directions

Mix the essential oil with the carrier oil and pour under running bath water.

March 20

Aromatic Oven Cleaner

Materials

- ½ cup unscented liquid soap

- 1 ½ cups baking soda

- ¼ cup vinegar

- 2 tsps. lemon

Directions

In a small bowl, mix all ingredients together until a paste forms. Use a brush to paint the interior of your oven with the paste, avoiding the heating elements. Close the oven door and wait for about 8 to 12 hours before removing paste. DO NOT TURN THE OVEN ON. Use a damp sponge to wipe the oven clean.

March 21

Aromatic Foaming Spring Hand Soap

Materials

- ¼ cup castile soap

- 1 tbsp. sweet almond oil

- 1 tbsp. vegetable glycerin

- Distilled water

- 12 drops vetiver

- 12 drops lemon

Directions

Add soap, almond oil, veggie glycerin, and essential oils to foaming soap bottle followed by the water. Stir with a wooden spoon, cap, and use.

March 22

Spring Love Potion Massage Oil

Materials

- 8 drops sandalwood
- 3 drops jasmine
- 2 drops vanilla
- 1-ounce carrier oil

Directions

Add all ingredients to a darkly colored bottle, cap, and shake.

March 23

Spring Hand Massage Oil

Materials

- 3 drops neroli
- 2 drops frankincense
- 2 drops bergamot
- 2 drops sweet orange
- 1 drop sandalwood
- 1-oince carrier oil

Directions

Add all ingredients to a darkly colored bottle, cap, and shake. Massage into hands as needed.

March 24

Spring Head Massage Oil

Materials

- 6 drops peppermint

- 3 drops rosemary

- 1-ounce carrier oil

Directions

Add all ingredients to a darkly colored bottle, cap, and shake. Massage ½ tsp. into temples and at the base of the neck.

March 25

Spring Nighttime Foot Massage Oil

Materials

- 1- drops Roman chamomile

- 1-ounce carrier oil

Directions

Add all ingredients to a darkly colored bottle, cap, and shake.

March 26

Love My Face Spring Massage Oil

Materials

- 3 drops frankincense

- 3 drops rose

- 2 drops geranium

- 2 drops carrot seed

- 1-ounce rosehip oil

Directions

Add all ingredients to a darkly colored bottle, cap, and shake. Massage a few drops into facial skin during nightly skincare routine.

March 27

Get Those Legs Going Massage Oil

Materials

- 4 drops juniper berry

- 2 drops grapefruit

- 1 drop cypress

- 1 drop lemon

- 1 drop sweet orange

- 1-ounce carrier oil

Directions

Add all ingredients to a darkly colored bottle, cap, and shake. This massage oil is great for diminishing cellulite.

March 28

I Love Spring Diffuser Oil Blend

Materials

- 2 drops geranium

- 3 drops lavender

- 3 drops roman chamomile

Directions

Add all essential oils to your diffuser.

March 29

Candy Shop Diffuser Oil Blend

Materials

- 4 drops wild orange

- 4 drops wintergreen

Directions

Add all essential oils to your diffuser.

March 30

Spring Forest Diffuser Oil Blend

Materials

- 2 drops lime

- 2 drops lemon

- 1 drop orange

- 1 drop bergamot

- 1 drop white fir

Directions

Add all essential oils to your diffuser.

March 31

So Fresh and So Clean Diffuser Oil Blend

Materials

- 4 drops vetiver

- 3 drops lemon

- 3 drops peppermint

Directions

Add all essential oils to your diffuser.

April

At last, Spring is here and in full swing! We've only scratched the surface in March's collection of Spring Fever aromatherapy recipes. This month we'll really take a dive into the diffuser blends that you can use to create a fresh, positive atmosphere within your home where you can stay focused, feel energized, and enjoy all of the spring sunshine.

April 1

Stay Focused Diffuser Oil Blend

Materials

- 2 drops wild orange
- 2 drops peppermint

Directions

Add all essential oils to your diffuser.

April 2

Citrus Overload Diffuser Oil Blend

Materials

- 2 drops lavender
- 2 drops lemon
- 2 drops rosemary

Directions

Add all essential oils to your diffuser.

April 3

Odor Buster Diffuser Oil Blend

Materials

- 2 drops lemon
- 2 drops tea tree
- 1 drop cilantro
- 1 drop lime

Directions

Add all essential oils to your diffuser.

April 4

Pretty Flowers Diffuser Oil Blend

Materials

- 1 drop geranium
- 2 drops lavender
- 2 drops roman chamomile

Directions

Add all essential oils to your diffuser.

April 5

Calm Down Diffuser Oil Blend

Materials

- 3 drops lavender

- 3 drops geranium

- 2 drops roman chamomile

- 2 drops clary sage

- 2 drops ylang ylang

Directions

Add all essential oils to your diffuser.

April 6

Grounding Diffuser Oil Blend

Materials

- 2 drops vetiver

- 2 drops cedarwood

Directions

Add all essential oils to your diffuser.

April 7

Slow Down Diffuser Oil Blend

Materials

- 4 drops cedarwood

- 3 drops lavender

Directions

Add all essential oils to your diffuser.

April 8

Set My Emotions Straight Diffuser Oil Blend

Materials

- 2 drops wild orange
- 2 drops bergamot
- 2 drops cypress
- 2 drops frankincense

Directions

Add all essential oils to your diffuser.

April 9

Color Me Happy Diffuser Oil Blend

Materials

- 2 drops lemon
- 2 drops wild orange
- 2 drops bergamot
- 2 drops grapefruit

Directions

Add all essential oils to your diffuser.

April 10

Wake Up, Honey Diffuser Oil Blend

Materials

- 4 drops wild orange
- 4 drops peppermint

Directions

Add all essential oils to your diffuser.

April 11

Little Piece of Sunshine Diffuser Oil Blend

Materials

- 3 drops wild orange
- 3 drops grapefruit
- 2 drops lemon
- 1 drop bergamot

Directions

Add all essential oils to your diffuser.

April 12

Energizer Bunny Diffuser Oil Blend

Materials

- 2 drops wild orange
- 2 drops frankincense
- 2 drops cinnamon

Directions

Add all essential oils to your diffuser.

April 13

Cool Down Diffuser Oil Blend

Materials

- 4 drops spearmint
- 4 drops peppermint
- 4 drops citronella
- 1 drop lemongrass

Directions

Add all essential oils to your diffuser.

April 14

Spring Sensation Diffuser Oil Blend

Materials

- 2 drops wild orange
- 2 drops jasmine
- 2 drops tangerine

Directions

Add all essential oils to your diffuser.

April 15

Spring Spark Diffuser Oil Blend

Materials

- 4 drops lavender

- 3 drops juniper berry

- 6 drops grapefruit

- 1 drop coriander

Directions

Add all essential oils to your diffuser.

April 16

Sugarcoated Spring Dreams Diffuser Oil Blend

Materials

- 6 drops cedarwood

- 4 drops lavender

- 3 drops tangerine

Directions

Add all essential oils to your diffuser.

April 17

Come Outside Diffuser Oil Blend

Materials

- 2 drops rose

- 2 drops geranium

- 2 drops helichrysum

Directions

Add all essential oils to your diffuser.

April 18

Dance With Me Diffuser Oil Blend

Materials

- 2 drops wild orange
- 2 drops ylang ylang
- 4 drops lemongrass

Directions

Add all essential oils to your diffuser.

April 19

Spring Hippie Diffuser Oil Blend

Materials

- 4 drops patchouli
- 2 drops sandalwood
- 2 drops cedarwood
- 1 drop lemongrass

Directions

Add all essential oils to your diffuser.

April 20

No More Stress Diffuser Oil Blend

Materials

- 2 drops bergamot
- 2 drops vanilla
- 1 drop lavender

Directions

Add all essential oils to your diffuser.

April 21

Anxiety Buster Diffuser Oil Blend

Materials

- 2 drops neroil
- 2 drops rose

Directions

Add all essential oils to your diffuser.

April 22

Spring Esteem Diffuser Oil Blend

Materials

- 2 drops cypress
- 2 drops jasmine
- 1 drop rosemary

Directions

Add all essential oils to your diffuser.

April 23

Stop Sadness Diffuser Oil Blend

Materials

- 4 drops bergamot

- 2 drops ylang ylang

- 2 drops clary sage

Directions

Add all essential oils to your diffuser.

April 24

Beat Spring Fatigue Diffuser Oil Blend

Materials

- 4 drops basil

- 2 drops peppermint

- 1 drop patchouli

Directions

Add all essential oils to your diffuser.

April 25

Calm My Agitated Soul Diffuser Oil Blend

Materials

- 2 drops roman chamomile
- 2 drops bergamot
- 1 drop lavender
- 1 drop mandarin
- 1 drop sandalwood

Directions

Add all essential oils to your diffuser.

April 26

Isolation Lifter Diffuser Oil Blend

Materials

- 2 drops frankincense
- 2 drops rose
- 1 drop roman chamomile

Directions

Add all essential oils to your diffuser.

April 27

Memory Booster Diffuser Oil Blend

Materials

- 2 drops basil
- 2 drops cypress
- 1 drop peppermint

- 1 drop rosemary

- 1 drop lemon

Directions

Add all essential oils to your diffuser.

April 28

Get Frisky Spring Diffuser Oil Blend

Materials

- 2 drops clary sage

- 2 drops ylang ylang

- 1 drop patchouli

- 1 drop vanilla

Directions

Add all essential oils to your diffuser.

April 29

Stay Balanced Diffuser Oil Blend

Materials

- 3 drops geranium

- 2 drops frankincense

- 1 drop bergamot

- 1 drop sandalwood

Directions

Add all essential oils to your diffuser.

April 30

Be Still My Heart Diffuser Oil Blend

Materials

- 2 drops lavender

- 2 drop vanilla

- 1 drop chamomile

Directions

Add all essential oils to your diffuser.

May

We all know that April showers bring May flowers, right? Right! During the month of May, we'll be focusing on floral aromatic blends for both the body and home. There's nothing more emotionally healing than the essence of floral blooms wafting under your nose.

May 1

Floral Carpet Deodorizer

Materials

- 50 drops lavender
- 1 cup baking soda

Directions

Mix the essential oil with the baking soda using a fork to evenly incorporate. Place the mixture in a shaker jar and spread over carpets and rugs. Allow to sit for at least 10 minutes before vacuuming.

May 2

Flowery Air Freshener

Materials

- 1 ½ oz. distilled water
- 1 ½ oz. vodka or witch hazel
- 10 drops geranium
- 10 drops rose
- 20 drops lavender

Directions

Mix water, oils, and vodka in a spray bottle, cap, and shake. Spray throughout your home.

May 3

Floral Room Spray

Materials

- 10 drops ylang ylang

- 6 drops rose

- 10 drops orange

- 4 drops cardamom

- 1 ½ oz. distilled water

- 1 ½ oz. vodka or witch hazel

Directions

Mix water, oils, and vodka in a spray bottle, cap, and shake. Spray throughout your home.

May 4

Earth Lover Room Spray

Materials

- 8 drops juniper berry

- 6 drops rosemary

- 4 drops frankincense

- 6 drops jasmine

- 1 ½ oz. distilled water

- 1 ½ oz. vodka or witch hazel

Directions

Mix water, oils, and vodka in a spray bottle, cap, and shake. Spray throughout your home.

May 5

Citrus Peels and Flowers Room Spray

Materials

- 10 drops lavender

- 8 drops sweet orange

- 4 drops bergamot

- 4 drops vanilla

- 1 ½ oz. distilled water

- 1 ½ oz. vodka or witch hazel

Directions

Mix water, oils, and vodka in a spray bottle, cap, and shake. Spray throughout your home.

May 6

Give Me Energy, Give Me Flowers Room Spray

Materials

- 20 drops lemon

- 8 drops eucalyptus

- 4 drops rose

- 2 drops cinnamon

- 2 drops peppermint

- 1 ½ oz. distilled water

- 1 ½ oz. vodka or witch hazel

Directions

Mix water, oils, and vodka in a spray bottle, cap, and shake. Spray throughout your home.

May 7

Aromatic Gel Air Freshener

Materials

- 1 packet Knox gelatin

- ¾ cup water

- ¼ cup vodka

- 7 drops lavender and 7 drops lemon (or your favorite essential oil scent)

- 2 drops food coloring

Directions

Bring the water to a boil in a small sauce pan and add in the gelatin. Stir until dissolved. Allow the mixture to cool to room temperature, then pour into a small jar followed by the vodka, essential oils, and food coloring. Stir and refrigerate. Remove from fridge when set.

May 8

Floral Sheet Spray

Materials

- 10 drops roman chamomile

- 10 drops geranium

- 5 drops lavender

- ½ cup. distilled water

- ½ cup vodka or witch hazel

Directions

Mix water, oils, and vodka in a spray bottle, cap, and shake. Spray on your sheets and other linens.

May 9

Scented Wax Sachets

Materials

- Wax paper

- Beeswax sheets or beeswax beads

- Stove pot

- Empty metal soup can

- Kitchen tongs

- Chopstick or wooden skewer

- 20 drops rose

- 20 drops lavender

- 10 drops sandalwood

- Fresh or dried flowers

- Soap mold

- Utility knife

- Lighter

- Long nail

- Jute Twine

Directions

Cover work surface with wax paper. Cut up the sheet of beeswax so they are small enough to fit inside of the soup can. Fill the pot with 1-inch of water and place the soup can inside. Turn the stove on medium-low heat. As the water starts to boil, hold the soup can with the tongs and place pieces of wax inside. As the wax begins to melt, stir it with the wooden skewer. Add essential oils to the melted wax and stir. Next, place the fresh or dried flowers into the soap mold. Remove wax mixture from heat and slowly pour into molds. Place additional flowers on top pf the wax. Place wax bars into the freezer for 20 minutes. Remove molds from freezer and flip upside down. The wax bars should come out of the molds. Remove excess wax from sides of bars with utility knife. Now, carefully heat the tip of the nail with a lighter. Pierce the hot nail through the corner of the wax bar making a hole. Threat the jute twine through the hole and tie. You can know hang your scented wax sachet anywhere you like.

May 10

Scented Toilet Paper

Materials

- 5 drops ylang ylang

Directions

Place a few drops of the essential oil inside of the cardboard toilet paper roll. Gives the bathroom a nice floral scent!

May 11

Aromatic Refrigerator Odor Buster

Materials

- 1 cup fresh or used coffee grounds

- 5 drops lemon

Directions

Place coffee grounds into a small bowl and add essential oil. Stir and place into the fridge overnight to bust odors. You can also make this recipe when wanting to remove odors from your kitchen by swapping out the lemon for lavender and placing the bowl on your countertop.

May 12

Floral Potpourri

Materials

- Dried strawberry slices

- Dried juniper berries

- Dried rose hips

- Dried rose petal

- Dried hibiscus flowers

- Dried lavender buds

- Pine cones

- 50 drops of your favorite floral essential oils

Directions

Add all ingredients to a large Ziploc bag, close, and shake. Pour the mixture into bowls or jars and set around your home for a pretty floral scent.

May 13

Fresh Aromatic Herb Bouquet

Materials

- Various herb clippings

- Wild Flowers

Directions

Create a bouquet using the materials listed and place in a vase on your dining room table to fill your home with a herbaceous floral scent.

May 14

Rosy Cheeks Face Cream

Materials

- 1 cup unscented lotion
- ¼ cup rose petal powder
- 5 drops rose EO

Directions

Mix all ingredients together and store in a glass jar. This crema can also be used on the body.

May 15

Rose Diffuser Blend

Materials

- 3 drops rose
- 1 drop geranium

Directions

Add essential oils to your diffuser.

May 16

Lavender Diffuser Blend

Materials

- 4 drops lavender

- 2 drops lemon

Directions

Add essential oils to your diffuser.

May 17

Roman Chamomile Diffuser Blend

Materials

- 6 drops roman chamomile

- 2 drops orange

Directions

Add essential oils to your diffuser.

May 18

Honey Suckle Diffuser Blend

Materials

- 5 drops honey suckle

- 2 drops vanilla

Directions

Add essential oils to your diffuser.

May 19

Clary Sage Diffuser Blend

Materials

- 3 drops clary sage
- 1 drop geranium
- 1 drop basil

Directions

Add essential oils to your diffuser.

May 20

Helichrysum Diffuser Blend

Materials

- 4 drops helichrysum
- 1 drop lavender

Directions

Add essential oils to your diffuser.

May 21

Lilac Diffuser Blend

Materials

- 6 drops lilac
- 1 drop lavender

Directions

Add essential oils to your diffuser.

May 22

Lilac Massage Oil

Materials

- 20 drops lavender

- 2 cups jojoba oil

Directions

Mix all ingredients and store in a glass jar.

May 23

Citrus Flower Massage Oil

Materials

- 2 drops clary sage

- 2 drops jasmine

- 12 drops bergamot

- 5 drops vanilla

- 3 drops ylang ylang

- 2 drops grapefruit

- 2 cups jojoba oil

Directions

Mix all ingredients and store in a glass jar.

May 24

Morning Blossom Massage Oil

Materials

- 3 drops ginger

- 3 drops cardamom

- 12 drops bergamot

- 5 drops frankincense

- 3 drops neroli

- 3 drops grapefruit

- 2 cups jojoba oil

Directions

Mix all ingredients and store in a glass jar.

May 25

Happy Hands Sanitizer

Materials

- ¼ cup aloe vera gel

- 20 drops orange

- 5 drops clove

- 10 drops cinnamon

- 10 drops lavender
- 5 drops rosemary

Directions

Mix all ingredients and store in a glass jar.

May 26

Aromatic Hair Gel

Materials

- ¼ tsp. unflavored gelatin
- ½ cup hot filtered water
- 6 drops lavender

Directions

Heat water and mix together with gelatin in a small bowl. Stir well to combine and refrigerate for about 3 hours, or until set. Once cooled and set, add essential oils if desired, and stir to combine. Using a funnel, transfer to a small squeeze bottle for easiest dispensing. Keep styling gel refrigerated between uses. Gel will keep for about 2 weeks in the refrigerator.

Source: http://www.diynatural.com/homemade-natural-hair-gel/

May 27

Aromatic Bubble Bath

Materials

- 1 cup castile soap

- ½ cup vegetable glycerin

- 2 tbsps. water

- 15 drops rose

Directions

Combine castile soap, glycerin, and water into a glass measuring cup. Add the essential oil and stir. Pour mixture into a glass jar and cap. Use ¼ cup per bath.

May 28

Floral Epsom Salt Bath

Materials

- 2 cup Epsom salts

- 20 drops lavender

Directions

Mix Epsom salts and essential oil together. Add scented salts to running tub water.

May 29

Lavender Foot Soak

Materials

- 1 cup Epsom salt

- 2 green tea bags

- 2 tsp. fresh or dried lavender buds

- ½ tsp. lavender essential oil

Directions

Mix all ingredients together and store in a mason jar. When ready to use, add mixture to a basin of hot water and soak feet.

May 30

Bedtime Flowers Diffuser Blend

Materials

- 4 drops lavender
- 2 drops rose
- 1 drop chamomile

Directions

Place all essential oil into your diffuser.

May 31

Nursery Diffuser Blend

Materials

- 1 drop lavender
- 1 drop chamomile
- 1 drop sweet orange

Directions

Place all essential oil into your diffuser.

June

Summer is finally here! How have you been enjoying your spring aromatherapy scents? I bet you are feeling revitalized and healthy. With summer comes a whole new ballgame of SCENTsational scents and aromatherapy blends. This chapter is all about summery scents and making you and your household feel great during the month of June.

June 1

Mountain Breeze Diffuser Blend

Materials

- 4 drops white fir
- 3 drops cedarwood
- 1 drop clove
- 1 drop peppermint

Directions

Place all essential oil into your diffuser.

June 2

By The Lake Diffuser Blend

Materials

- 3 drops lavender
- 3 drops grapefruit
- 3 drops lemon

- 2 drops spearmint

Directions

Place all essential oil into your diffuser.

June 3

Seashore Diffuser Blend

Materials

- 1 drop vetiver
- 2 drops lavender
- 3 drops bergamot

Directions

Place all essential oil into your diffuser.

June 4

Summer In Italy Diffuser Blend

Materials

- 3 drops bergamot
- 3 drops lemon
- 3 drops cypress

Directions

Place all essential oil into your diffuser.

June 5

Summer Snoozin' Diffuser Blend

Materials

- 2 drops lavender

- 2 drops wild orange

- 2 drops sandalwood

Directions

Place all essential oil into your diffuser.

June 6

Adventurous Mood Diffuser Blend

Materials

- 2 drops basil

- 1 drop cypress

- 2 drops grapefruit

Directions

Place all essential oil into your diffuser.

June 7

Summer Meditation Diffuser Blend

Materials

- 1 drop vetiver

- 2 drops cedarwood

- 1 drop sandalwood

- 2 drops wild orange

- 3 drops lavender

Directions

Place all essential oil into your diffuser.

June 8

Summer Restoration Diffuser Blend

Materials

- 2 drops frankincense

- 2 drops juniper berry

- 2 drops bergamot

Directions

Place all essential oil into your diffuser.

June 9

Set My Soul Free Diffuser Blend

Materials

- 3 drops grapefruit

- 3 drops eucalyptus

- 2 drops peppermint

Directions

Place all essential oil into your diffuser.

June 10

Clean Abode Diffuser Blend

Materials

- 3 drops lemon

- 3 drops orange

Directions

Place all essential oil into your diffuser.

June 11

Summer Stress Relief Diffuser Blend

Materials

- 2 drops bergamot

- 2 drops rosemary

- 1 drop white fir

- 2 drops peppermint

Directions

Place all essential oil into your diffuser.

June 12

Summer Spa Retreat Diffuser Blend

Materials

- 1 drop geranium
- 3 drops lavender
- 4 drops lime

Directions

Place all essential oil into your diffuser.

June 13

Summer at Dusk Diffuser Blend

Materials

- 4 drops juniper berry
- 2 drops grapefruit
- 3 drops bergamot
- 1 drop ylang ylang

Directions

Place all essential oil into your diffuser.

June 14

Wake Up Sleepy Head Diffuser Blend

Materials

- 1 drop lemon
- 1 drop orange
- 1 drop lime
- 1 drop grapefruit
- 3 drops peppermint

Directions

Place all essential oil into your diffuser.

June 15

Summer Heat Buster Diffuser Blend

Materials

- 3 drops lavender
- 3 drops peppermint

Directions

Place all essential oil into your diffuser.

June 16

Summer Declutter Diffuser Blend

Materials

- 2 drops sandalwood
- 3 drops lemon

- 2 drops orange

Directions

Place all essential oil into your diffuser.

June 17

Feel Safe Summer Diffuser Blend

Materials

- 3 drops juniper berry

- 2 drops lavender

- 2 drops chamomile

Directions

Place all essential oil into your diffuser.

June 18

Bottoms Up Diffuser Blend

Materials

- 3 drops bergamot

- 2 drops grapefruit

- 2 drops cypress

- 2 drops frankincense

- 1 drop ylang ylang

- 1 drop ginger

Directions

Place all essential oil into your diffuser.

June 19

Summer Health Diffuser Blend

Materials

- 1 drop tea tree

- 2 drops lemon

- 3 drops wild orange

Directions

Place all essential oil into your diffuser.

June 20

Late Night At The Office Diffuser Blend

Materials

- 4 drops lemon

- 3 drops basil

- 2 drops rosemary

- 2 drops cypress

- 1 drop peppermint

Directions

Place all essential oil into your diffuser.

June 21

Summer Weekend Diffuser Blend

Materials

- 3 drops white fir

- 3 drops geranium

- 2 drops lemongrass

- 1 drop cypress

- 1 drop grapefruit

Directions

Place all essential oil into your diffuser.

June 22

Summer Rain Diffuser Blend

Materials

- 3 drops bergamot

- 2 drops lavender

- 2 drops clary sage

Directions

Place all essential oil into your diffuser.

June 23

Yoga Diffuser Blend

Materials

- 4 drops orange

- 2 drops patchouli

- 2 drops Indian neroli

- 1 drop champa

- 1 drop rosewood

Directions

Place all essential oil into your diffuser.

June 24

Mountain Breeze Diffuser Blend

Materials

- 3 drops frankincense

- 3 drops lavender

- 2 drops bergamot

Directions

Place all essential oil into your diffuser.

June 25

Peaceful Little One Diffuser Blend

Materials

- 4 drops vetiver
- 3 drops ylang ylang
- 2 drops frankincense
- 1 drop clary sage
- 1 drop marjoram

Directions

Place all essential oil into your diffuser.

June 26

Summer Workout Diffuser Blend

Materials

- 2 drops lemon
- 2 drops lime
- 3 drops grapefruit

Directions

Place all essential oil into your diffuser.

June 27

Summer Snuggles Diffuser Blend

Materials

- 3 drops lavender
- 3 drops ylang ylang
- 3 drops sandalwood

Directions

Place all essential oil into your diffuser.

June 28

Summer Stink Buster Diffuser Blend

Materials

- 2 drops lemon
- 1 drop tea tree
- 1 drop cilantro
- 1 drop lime

Directions

Place all essential oil into your diffuser.

June 29

Moonlit Path Diffuser Blend

Materials

- 3 drops cedarwood

- 3 drops juniper berry

- 2 drops cypress

- 1 drop lime

Directions

Place all essential oil into your diffuser.

June 30

Summer Friendship Diffuser Blend

Materials

- 6 drops cinnamon

- 2 drops frankincense

- 1 drop ginger

- 1 drop lemon

Directions

Place all essential oil into your diffuser.

July

Summer is in full swing and so is your life! Just because it's summer doesn't mean that life slows down. Between picnics, parties, BBQs, and vacations, you need a little rest and restoration. This chapter focuses on aromatic blends that will bring joy, peace, and comfort to your life during the busy summer month of July. You might even find a bug repellent recipe or two hiding in the mix.

July 1

Bugs Be Gone Diffuser Blend

Materials

- 3 drops lavender
- 2 drops white fir
- 1 drop peppermint

Directions

Place all essential oil into your diffuser.

July 2

Summer Slumber Diffuser Blend

Materials

- 4 drops lavender
- 3 drops vetiver

Directions

Place all essential oil into your diffuser.

July 3

Hanging Out at Home Diffuser Blend

Materials

- 4 drops chamomile
- 2 drops valerian
- 1 drop tangerine

Directions

Place all essential oil into your diffuser.

July 4

Relax On My Lap Diffuser Blend

Materials

- 3 drops lavender
- 2 drops cedarwood

Directions

Place all essential oil into your diffuser.

July 5

Sweet Summer Daydreams Diffuser Blend

Materials

- 3 drops ylang ylang
- 2 drops cedarwood

- 2 drops marjoram

Directions

Place all essential oil into your diffuser.

July 6

Naptime Diffuser Blend

Materials

- 5 drops lavender

- 2 drops frankincense

Directions

Place all essential oil into your diffuser.

July 7

Sleepy Smiles Diffuser Blend

Materials

- 2 drops frankincense

- 2 drops chamomile

- 2 drops cedarwood

Directions

Place all essential oil into your diffuser.

July 8

Happy Dreams Diffuser Blend

Materials

- 2 drops cinnamon
- 1 drop clove
- 1 drop lavender
- 3 drops valerian

Directions

Place all essential oil into your diffuser.

July 9

Insect Blaster Aromatic Spray

Materials

- 2 tbsps. witch hazel
- 2 tbsps. grapeseed oil
- ½ tsp. vodka
- 55 drops eucalyptus
- 15 drops cedarwood
- 15 drops lavender
- 15 drops rosemary

Direction

Place all carrier liquids in a small spray bottle followed by essential oils. Cap and shake. Apply to clothing, exposed skin, and surroundings every few hours when bugs are a problem.

July 10

Aerobics Time Diffuser Blend

Materials

- 2 drops spearmint

- 2 drops tangerine

- 2 drops lemon

Directions

Place all essential oil into your diffuser.

July 11

Staycation Diffuser Blend

Materials

- 3 drops rosemary

- 3 drops bergamot

Directions

Place all essential oil into your diffuser.

July 12

Exotic Vacation Diffuser Blend

Materials

- 10 drops patchouli
- 3 drops orange
- 2 drops ylang ylang

Directions

Place all essential oil into your diffuser.

July 13

Summer Sweetie Diffuser Blend

Materials

- 4 drops tangerine
- 2 drops lavender
- 1 drop lime
- 1 drop spearmint

Directions

Place all essential oil into your diffuser.

July 14

Sunshiny Day Diffuser Blend

Materials

- 2 drops wild orange
- 2 drops grapefruit
- 2 drops clove
- 2 drops lemon
- 1 drop wintergreen

Directions

Place all essential oil into your diffuser.

July 15

Tahitian Vacation Diffuser Blend

Materials

- 3 drops wild orange
- 2 drops ginger
- 2 drops ylang ylang

Directions

Place all essential oil into your diffuser.

July 16

Alpine Dreams On A Summer Day Diffuser Blend

Materials

- 2 drops bergamot

- 1 drop cedarwood

- 2 drops wintergreen

Directions

Place all essential oil into your diffuser.

July 17

Jet Lag Morning Mist

Materials

- 2 drops basil

- 2 drops peppermint

- 2 drops lemon

- 1 oz. purified water

Directions

Place all essential oils and water into a small spray bottle, cap, shake, and spray.

July 18

Jet Lag Evening Mist

Materials

- 2 drops geranium

- 2 drops sweet marjoram

- 2 drops lavender

- 1 oz. purified water

Directions

Place all essential oils and water into a small spray bottle, cap, shake, and spray.

July 19

Bugs Be Gone Diffuser Blend

Materials

- 3 drops lavender

- 2 drops white fir

- 1 drop peppermint

Directions

Place all essential oil into your diffuser.

July 20

You're getting On My Nerves Diffuser Blend

Materials

- 2 drops lavender

- 2 drops wild orange

- 1 drop geranium

- 1 drop clary sage

Directions

Place all essential oil into your diffuser.

July 21

Island Vacation Diffuser Blend

Materials

- 1 drop orange
- 1 drop lemon
- 1 drop grapefruit
- 1 drop lime
- 2 drops ylang ylang
- 2 drops jasmin

Directions

Place all essential oil into your diffuser.

July 22

Get Herbal Summer Diffuser Blend

Materials

- 1 drop basil
- 1 drop geranium
- 2 drops frankincense

Directions

Place all essential oil into your diffuser.

July 23

Aromatic Car Diffuser Blend

Materials

- 3 drops wild orange
- 3 drops wintergreen

Directions

Place all essential oil into your car diffuser.

July 24

Get Up and Get Stuff Done Diffuser Blend

Materials

- 4 drops spearmint
- 2 drops peppermint
- 4 drops tangerine

Directions

Place all essential oil into your diffuser.

July 25

Mojito Diffuser Blend

Materials

- 2 drops peppermint
- 5 drops lime

Directions

Place all essential oil into your diffuser.

July 26

I Am Woman Summer Blend Diffuser Blend

Materials

- 3 drops lavender
- 3 drops clary sage
- 2 drops geranium
- 2 drops palmarosa

Directions

Place all essential oil into your diffuser.

July 27

Summer Treehouse Diffuser Blend

Materials

- 2 drops lavender

- 2 drops ylang ylang

- 2 drops tangerine

- 1 drop vanilla

Directions

Place all essential oil into your diffuser.

July 28

Cali Coast Diffuser Blend

Materials

- 1 drop rosemary

- 2 drops wild orange

- 2 drops cedarwood

- 2 drops frankincense

Directions

Place all essential oil into your diffuser.

July 29

Summer Date Night Gone Diffuser Blend

Materials

- 2 drops cinnamon bark

- 2 drops patchouli

- 2 drops rosemary

- 6 drops sandalwood

- 2 drops ylang ylang

Directions

Place all essential oil into your diffuser.

July 30

Summer Clover Patch Diffuser Blend

Materials

- 2 drops rosemary

- 2 drops spearmint

- 1 drop orange

Directions

Place all essential oil into your diffuser.

July 31

Summer Morning Cinnamon Bun Diffuser Blend

Materials

- 2 drops wild orange

- 2 drops cardamom

- 2 drops cassia

Directions

Place all essential oil into your diffuser.

August

Here we find ourselves at the tail end of summer. It always goes by so fast, doesn't it? Before you know it the kids will be back in school, you'll be back to work, and your routine will make the transition from summer fun to the hustle and bustle of life again. Let's make this transition smooth by kissing summer goodbye with soothing aromatherapy blends. Welcome to August.

August 1

Zippy Diffuser Blend

Materials

- 2 drops lemongrass
- 1 drop ginger

Directions

Place all essential oil into your diffuser.

August 2

Sunday Brunch Diffuser Blend

Materials

- 2 drops black pepper
- 1 drop ylang ylang
- 2 drops orange

Directions

Place all essential oil into your diffuser.

August 3

Chill Out, Dude Diffuser Blend

Materials

- 3 drops grapefruit
- 3 drops tangerine
- 2 drops lime
- 1 drop bergamot

Directions

Place all essential oil into your diffuser.

August 4

Feeling Grateful Diffuser Blend

Materials

- 2 drops orange
- 4 drops bergamot
- 2 drops geranium
- 2 drops white fir

Directions

Place all essential oil into your diffuser.

August 5

Summer Men's Diffuser Blend

Materials

- 2 drops white fir
- 2 drops rosemary
- 2 drops cypress
- 2 drops wintergreen

Directions

Place all essential oil into your diffuser.

August 6

Summer Refresher Diffuser Blend

Materials

- 6 drops pink grapefruit
- 6 drops petitgrian
- 3 drops rosemary

Directions

Place all essential oil into your diffuser.

August 7

Feeling Manly Diffuser Blend

Materials

- 1 drop bergamot
- 1 drop cypress
- 1 drop arborvitae

Directions

Place all essential oil into your diffuser.

August 8

Lucky Loo Diffuser Blend

Materials

- 2 drops white fir
- 3 drops arborvitae
- 1 drop lime

Directions

Place all essential oil into your diffuser.

August 9

Well of Joy Blend

Materials

- 2 drops geranium
- 3 drops lavender
- 4 drops lime

Directions

Place all essential oil into your diffuser.

August 10

Sittin' In My Hammock Diffuser Blend

Materials

- 3 drops lavender

- 3 drops clary sage

- 3 drops lime

Directions

Place all essential oil into your diffuser.

August 11

Happy Children Diffuser Blend

Materials

- 2 drops frankincense

- 2 drops spearmint

- 2 drops lime

- 2 drops sweet orange

Directions

Place all essential oil into your diffuser.

August 12

Coconut Oil Salt Scrub

Materials

- 1 cup fractionated coconut oil

- ½ cup Epsom salts

- 10 drops lime EO

Directions

Mix coconut oil with Epsom salts followed by essential oil. Place into a glass jar and use in the shower.

August 13

Scalp Awakening Aromatic Oil

Materials

- 2 tbsps. coconut oil, melted

- 1 drop lemon EO

Directions

Mix essential oil with coconut oil and massage into scalp. Allow to sit on scalp for 30 minutes. Shampoo as normal.

August 14

Aromatic Lime, Basil, and Mandarin Room Spray

Materials

- 2 oz. distilled water

- 1 oz. vodka

- 10 drops basil

- 10 drops lime

- 10 drops mandarin

Directions

Place water and vodka into a fine mister spray bottle followed by essential oils, cap, and shake.

August 15

So Long Summer Diffuser Blend

Materials

- 2 drops lemon

- 2 drops lime

- 1 drop vanilla

Directions

Place all essential oil into your diffuser.

August 16

Summer Pet Spray

Materials

- 2 drops peppermint EO
- ¼ tsp. clear vanilla extract
- ¼ tsp. argan oil
- 2 oz. water

Directions

Place argan oil, essential oil, and vanilla into a 2.5 oz. spray bottle, cap, and shake. Open the bottle and add the water, cap, and shake. Spray on dog as needed, avoiding the eyes and face.

August 17

Any Day Diffuser Blend

Materials

- 2 drops lemon
- 1 drop lavender

Directions

Place all essential oil into your diffuser.

August 18

Aromatic Cuticle cream

Materials

- 1 ½ oz, beeswax pellets
- 3 oz. apricot kernel oil

- 1 tbsps. raw honey

- 5 drops lavender EO

Directions

Place the beeswax, apricot oil, and honey into a glass bowl and micro-wave in 15-second intervals until melted. Stir between intervals. Add essential oil to wax mixture and store in a small tin or glass baby food jar. Massage into cuticles as needed.

August 19

Aromatic Toenail Cuticle Oil

Materials

- 2 tbsps. coconut oil

- 1 drop tea tree EO

- 2 drops lavender EO

Directions

Mix all oils together and rub onto toes. This is a great aromatherapy recipe for killing fungus and bacteria.

August 20

Midnight Bliss Diffuser Blend

Materials

- 2 drops lavender

- 2 drops vanilla

- 1 drops jasmin

Directions

Place all essential oil into your diffuser.

August 21

Relief Diffuser Blend

Materials

- 3 drops lavender

- 3 drops lime

- 3 drops mandarin

Directions

Place all essential oil into your diffuser.

August 22

Jump Up and Down Diffuser Blend

Materials

- 3 drops orange

- 3 drops frankincense

- 2 drops cinnamon

Directions

Place all essential oil into your diffuser.

August 23

Healthy Bodies Blend

Materials

- 3 drops lemon

- 2 drops oregano

Directions

Place all essential oil into your diffuser.

August 24

Time for Bed Diffuser Blend

Materials

- 3 drops juniper berry

- 3 drops roman chamomile

- 3 drops lavender

Directions

Place all essential oil into your diffuser.

August 25

Summer Headache Go Away Diffuser Blend

Materials

- 6 drops peppermint

- 4 drops eucalyptus

- 2 drops myrrh

Directions

Place all essential oil into your diffuser.

August 26

Get Out of My Life Bugs Diffuser Blend

Materials

- 4 drops spearmint
- 4 drops peppermint
- 4 drops citronella
- 1 drop lemongrass

Directions

Place all essential oil into your diffuser.

August 27

Buggy Buster Diffuser Blend

Materials

- 2 drops lemongrass
- 2 drops thyme
- 2 drops eucalyptus
- 2 drops basil

Directions

Place all essential oil into your diffuser.

August 28

Welcome to My Summer Cottage Diffuser Blend

Materials

- 3 drops lavender
- 3 drops lemon
- 3 drops rosemary

Directions

Place all essential oil into your diffuser.

August 29

Fresh Forest Diffuser Blend

Materials

- 4 drops frankincense
- 3 drops white fir
- 2 drops cedarwood

Directions

Place all essential oil into your diffuser.

August 30

Summer Romance Diffuser Blend

Materials

- 3 drops grapefruit
- 3 drops lavender
- 2 drops lemon
- 2 drops spearmint
- 1 drop vanilla

Directions

Place all essential oil into your diffuser.

August 31

Farewell to Thee, Summer Diffuser Blend

Materials

- 4 drops wild orange
- 3 drops cinnamon
- 2 drops clove

Directions

Place all essential oil into your diffuser.

September

Summer has left us, folks. Until next year, we bid farewell to thee, sweet Summer. However, there's nothing to be sad about because with September comes the wonderful Fall season. Cozy, crackling fires, apple cider, falling leaves, and so many more things to be excited about. Aromatherapy blends for the fall will certainly put a smile on your face! This month we focus on diffuser blends that bring about focus, clarity, and peace of mind when going back to school, work, and creating new projects.

September 1

Wake Up for School Diffuser Blend

Materials

- 2 drops wild orange
- 2 drops peppermint
- 1 drop oregano

Directions

Place all essential oil into your diffuser.

September 2

Remember What You Learned Diffuser Blend

Materials

- 2 drops rosemary
- 2 drops lemon
- 1 drop spearmint

Directions

Place all essential oil into your diffuser.

September 3

Protect My Health, Mom Diffuser Blend

Materials

- 3 drops Thieves blend by Young Living Oils

Directions

Place all essential oil into your diffuser.

September 4

Stay Calm During That Test Diffuser Blend

Materials

- 2 drops lavender
- 2 drops roman chamomile
- 1 drop ginger

Directions

Place all essential oil into your diffuser.

September 5

Happy Yummy Diffuser Blend

Materials

- 2 drops ginger
- 1 drop peppermint
- 1 drop lemon

Directions

Place all essential oil into your diffuser.

September 6

Aromatic Acne Buster Face Wash

Materials

- ¼ cup castile soap
- ¼ cup brewed organic chamomile tea
- ¾ tsp. grapeseed oil
- 6 drops lemon EO
- 2 drops tea tree EO
- 4 drops vitamin E oil

Directions

Brew a cup of chamomile tea and allow ¼ of it to cool. While waiting, mix all other ingredients together in a small bowl, then add the tea and stir. Pour face wash into a squirt bottle and keep closed tightly. Use on face as you normally would any other cleanser.

September 7

Aromatic Solution for A Stinky Backpack

Materials

- 1 cotton ball
- 1 drop essential oil

Directions

Using your favorite essential oil, place one drop onto a cotton ball and toss into your backpack to snuff out unpleasant odors.

September 8

Aromatic Armpit Odor Buster

Materials

- ½ cup cornstarch
- ½ cup baking soda
- 20 drops lavender EO
- 10 drops patchouli EO

Directions

Mix all ingredients together in a glass jar and stir with a fork. Dust armpits with the powder to prevent odor. Keep jar tightly closed between uses.

September 9

Dorm Room Deodorizer

Materials

- ½ cup white vinegar

- 5 drops essential oil

- Small bowl

Directions

Place all vinegar and your favorite essential oils into a small bowl and set out in the corner of your room to bust nasty smells. Make sure no pets are bale to drink the mixture.

September 10

Stop Stinking Up My Space, Puppy Dog

Materials

- 1 charcoal briquette

- 5 drops essential oil

Directions

Place the essential oil of your choice on the charcoal briquette and leave it in the corner of the room your pet is stinking up.

September 11

College Kid Car Deodorizer

Materials

- 1 oz. vodka

- 2 oz. distilled water

- 20 drops favorite essential oil

Directions

Mix all ingredients into a spray bottle, cap, and shake. Always shake well before spraying solution onto interior fabric of the car.

September 12

Freshen Up Furniture Spray

Materials

- 1 oz. vodka

- 2 oz. distilled water

- 1 tbsps. baking soda

- 20 drops orange EO

- 5 drops rosemary EO

Directions

Place baking soda and essential oils into a bowl and stir with a fork. Add vodka and water to a spray bottle. Using a funnel, add the baking soda mixture to the bottle, cap, and shake. Spray on musty furniture, carpets, and curtains to freshen them up.

September 13

Frat Boy Freezer Freshener

Materials

- 1 clean sock

- 1 cup coffee grounds

- 5 drops lemon EO

Directions

Place coffee into a small bowl followed by the essential oil. Stir together with a fork, and place the mixture into the clean sock. Tie the sock closed and place into the freezer to absorb foul odors.

September 14

Instant Classroom Calmer Diffuser Blend

Materials

- 5 drops bergamot

Directions

Place all essential oil into your diffuser.

September 15

Calming Aromatherapy Rice Box

Materials

- 1 small wooden trinket box

- 1-2 cups uncooked rice

- 1 handful of marbles

- 10 drops lavender EO

Directions

Place the rice and marbles into a Ziploc bag followed by the essential oil. Closed the bag and shake. Pour the mixture into the box. When children (and adults) seem anxious or tense, allow them to run their hands through the box to "play" with the rice and marbles while experiencing the calming aromatic benefits of lavender.

September 16

Natural Classroom Air Freshener

Materials

- 1 pint-sized glass jar

- Small square of fabric

- Jar ring

- 1 cup baking soda

- 20 drops essential oil

Directions

Place baking soda and essential oils of your choice into the jar and stir with a fork. Put the square of fabric on the jar's opening and secure with the ring. Place in the classroom to keep smells at bay.

September 17

Aromatic Cloud Dough

Materials

- 8 cups flour

- 1 cup vegetable oil

- 5 drops lavender EO

Directions

Mix all materials together in a bowl and transfer to an airtight container. You may color the dough with a bit of powdered tempera paint or crushed chalk is you want. Allow children to mold the cloud dough with their hands and experience aromatherapy as they do so.

September 18

Aromatic Plant Therapy

Materials

- Flowering plant of your choice

Directions

Place plant on your desk or windowsill to experience it's floral essence and amazing oxygenating properties while you work or study.

September 19

Study Time Diffuser Blend

Materials

- 2 drops vetiver
- 3 drops Valor Blend by Young Living Oils

Directions

Place all essential oil into your diffuser.

September 20

Concentration Diffuser Blend

Materials

- 2 drops lemon
- 2 drops Hyssop

Directions

Place all essential oil into your diffuser.

September 21

Wrap Your Mind Around Your Work Diffuser Blend

Materials

- 2 drops peppermint
- 3 drops orange

Directions

Place all essential oil into your diffuser.

September 22

I Want to Learn Diffuser Blend

Materials

- 2 drops lavender
- 1 drop rosemary
- 1 drop cinnamon
- 2 drops lemon

Directions

Place all essential oil into your diffuser.

September 23

Reading Nook Diffuser Blend

Materials

- 3 drops peppermint
- 2 drops cinnamon
- 1 drop rosemary

Directions

Place all essential oil into your diffuser.

September 24

School is Cool Diffuser Blend

Materials

- 1 drop rosemary

- 2 drops peppermint

- 2 drops frankincense

Directions

Place all essential oil into your diffuser.

September 25

Before School Diffuser Blend

Materials

- 4 drops cypress

- 1 drop peppermint

Directions

Place all essential oil into your diffuser.

September 26

Take to School Aromatic Roller Blend

Materials

- 2 drops wild orange

- 2 drops lemon

- 1 drop rosemary

- 2 tbsps. fractionated coconut oil

Directions

Place essential oils and coconut oil into a small bowl and mix. Using a small funnel, pour the oil into a roller ball container and cap. Instruct children to use the roller ball aromatherapy mixture during the day at school as needed.

September 27

Go Away College Cootie Diffuser Blend

Materials

- 2 drops orange

- 2 drops clove

- 2 drops cinnamon

- 2 drops eucalyptus

- 2 drops rosemary

Directions

Place all essential oil into your diffuser.

September 28

Soothing Sugar Scrub Blend

Materials

- 1 cup white sugar

- ½ cup almond oil

- 10 drops orange EO

Directions

Mix all ingredients together and store in a glass jar. Use in the shower to scrub away the stresses of your busy life.

September 29

Grumpy Kids Be Gone Diffuser Blend

Materials

- 2 drops Peace and Calming by Young Living Oils

Directions

Place all essential oil into your diffuser.

September 30

Bake My Bad Mood Away (Cinnamon Rolls)

Materials

- 1 packet instant yeast

- 1 cup unsweetened plain almond milk

- ½ cup butter

- ¼ tsp. salt

- 3 cups flour

- 1 ½ tsp. ground cinnamon

- ¼ cup + 1 tbsp. can sugar, divided

Directions

Nothing beats the morning blues like fresh cinnamon rolls baking in the oven does! Even foods can give us a healthy does of much needed aromatherapy.

1. In a large sauce pan (or in a bowl in the microwave at 30 sec increments), heat the almond milk and 3 Tbsp Earth Balance until warm and melted, never reaching boiling. Remove from heat and let cool to 110 degrees F (43 C), or the temperature of bath water. It should be warm but not too hot or it will kill the yeast.

2. Transfer mixture to a large mixing bowl and sprinkle on yeast. Let activate for 10 minutes, then add 1 Tbsp sugar and the salt and stir.

3. Next add in flour 1/2 cup (68 g) at a time, stirring as you go. The dough will be sticky. When it is too thick to stir, transfer to a lightly floured surface and knead for a minute or so until it forms a loose ball. Rinse your mixing bowl out, coat it with canola or grapeseed oil, and add your dough ball back in. Cover with plastic wrap and set in a warm place to rise for about 1 hour, or until doubled in size.

4. On a lightly floured surface, roll out the dough into a thin rectangle. Brush with 3 Tbsp melted Earth Balance and top with 1/4 cup sugar and 1/2 - 1 Tbsp cinnamon (to taste).

5. Starting at one end, tightly roll up the dough and situate seam side down. Then with a serrated knife or a string of floss, cut the dough into 1.5 - 2 inch sections and position in a well-buttered 8x8-inch square or comparable sized round pan (you should have about 10 rolls). Brush with remaining 2 Tbsp Earth Balance (melted) and

cover with plastic wrap. Set on top of the oven to let rise again while you preheat oven to 350 degrees F (176 C).

6. Once the oven is hot, bake rolls for 25-30 minutes or until slightly golden brown. Let cool for a few minutes and then serve immediately.

Source: http://minimalistbaker.com/the-worlds-easiest-cinnamon-rolls/

October

Hello, Fall! The autumn season is officially in full swing and with it comes amazingly spicy aromatherapy scents for the diffuser. In addition to be known for scents like cinnamon, nutmeg, and apple, October is also home to many pumpkin scents in recognition of the spooky holiday known as, Halloween. So, straighten your witch's hat, fire up your diffuser, and get ready to experience the many aromatherapy blends that this great fall month has to offer.

October 1

Pumpkin Pie Diffuser Blend

Materials

- 5 drops cinnamon
- 1 drop clove
- 1 drop nutmeg

Directions

Place all essential oil into your diffuser.

October 2

Autumn Spice Diffuser Blend

Materials

- 4 drops orange
- 3 drops ginger
- 2 drops cinnamon

Directions

Place all essential oil into your diffuser.

October 3

Spiced Chai Diffuser Blend

Materials

- 3 drops cardamom
- 2 drops cinnamon
- 2 drops clove
- 1 drop ginger

Directions

Place all essential oil into your diffuser.

October 4

Walk in the Autumn Woods Diffuser Blend

Materials

- 3 drops frankincense
- 2 drops fir
- 1 drop cedarwood

Directions

Place all essential oil into your diffuser.

October 5

Fall Family Hike Diffuser Blend

Materials

- 4 drops cypress
- 2 drops fir
- 2 drops sandalwood

Directions

Place all essential oil into your diffuser.

October 6

Falling Leaves Diffuser Blend

Materials

- 5 drops orange
- 1 drop patchouli
- 1 drop ginger

Directions

Place all essential oil into your diffuser.

October 7

Spicy citrus Diffuser Blend

Materials

- 3 drops wild orange

- 2 drops cinnamon bark
- 1 drop clove

Directions

Place all essential oil into your diffuser.

October 8

Fall Sniffle Snuffer Diffuser Blend

Materials

- 1 drop rosemary
- 1 drop clove
- 1 drop eucalyptus
- 1 drop cinnamon bark
- 1 drop orange

Directions

Place all essential oil into your diffuser.

October 9

Autumn Air Diffuser Blend

Materials

- 4 drops sweet orange
- 3 drops lemon
- 3 drops fir

Directions

Place all essential oil into your diffuser.

October 10

Spicy Cinnamon Diffuser Blend

Materials

- 2 drops orange
- 1 drop cinnamon bark
- 1 drop clove
- 1 drop vanilla

Directions

Place all essential oil into your diffuser.

October 11

Fall Wreath Diffuser Blend

Materials

- 3 drops peppermint
- 3 drops fir
- 1 drop eucalyptus
- 1 drop tea tree
- 2 drops rosemary

Directions

Place all essential oil into your diffuser.

October 12

Aromatic Autumn Perfume Blend

Materials

- 12-20 drops base essential oils like cedarwood, vanilla, vetiver, ylang ylang, or sandalwood

- 1 tsp. vanilla extract

- 25-30 drops middle tone essential oils like rose, lavender, chamomile, or geranium

- 12-15 drops top note essential oils like bergamot, orange, or neroli

- 4 oz. spiced rum

Directions

Mix all oils together in a opaque bottle, cap, and allow the oils to mingle together for a day or two. Then, add the spiced rum and cap tightly. Shake and put the perfume in a cool, dark place for a t least 1 month before using.

October 13

Fall Essential Oil Diffuser Necklace

Materials

- 1 diffuser necklace

- 1 drop cinnamon bark

- 1 drop orange

- 1 drops vanilla

Directions

Place all essential oils onto the pad of the diffuser necklace and wear around your neck.

October 14

Pumpkin spice Sugar Scrub

Materials

- 1 ¾ cup brown sugar

- ¼ cup white sugar

- 1 drop cinnamon leaf

- 1 drop clove

- 1 drop ginger

- 1 drop nutmeg

- ¼ cup almond oil

- 1 tbsp. raw honey

Directions

Combine all sugars in a mixing bowl. Mix the oils and honey together in a separate bowl. Combine the liquid mixture with the sugars in a bowl and stir. Transfer to a mason jar for storing.

October 15

Aromatic Autumn Potpourri Blend

Materials

- Dried apple slices
- Dried orange slices
- Whole nuts with their shells
- Cinnamon sticks
- Whole cloves
- Juniper berries
- Dried rose hips
- Laurel (bay) leaves
- Pine Cones
- 10 drops cedarwood
- 10 drops clove
- 10 drops cinnamon
- 10 drops orange
- 10 drops pine

Directions

Place all ingredients into a large Ziploc bag, close, and shake. You can allow the bag to sit closed overnight for a stronger scent or immediately disperse the potpourri to jars or bowls around your home.

October 16

Fall Pot Simmer

Materials

- 1-quart water

- 4-5 laurel (bay) leaves

- 1 small orange, thinly sliced

- 1 large sprig of fresh rosemary

- 1 vanilla bean or 1-2 tsps. Vanilla extract

Directions

Place all ingredients into a saucepan and cover with water. Turn the heat on to medium-high. Allow mixture to simmer for 15-20 minutes, or more to make the home smell like a fresh fall day.

October 17

Autumn Room Mist

Materials

- 3 tbsps. vodka

- 10 drops juniper berry

- 10 drops clary sage

- 10 drops bergamot

- 10 drops cinnamon bark

Directions

Combine all ingredients into a spray bottle, cap, and shake. Spray around your home for an aromatic autumn experience.

October 18

Woodsy, Fall Room Mist

Materials

- 3 tbsps. vodka
- 10 drops cedarwood
- 10 drops rosemary
- 10 drops orange
- 10 drops clove

Directions

Combine all ingredients into a spray bottle, cap, and shake. Spray around your home for an aromatic woodsy fall experience.

October 19

Vanilla Passion Diffuser Blend

Materials

- 5 drops vanilla
- 3 drops lemon
- 1 drop rosemary

Directions

Add all essential oil to your diffuser.

October 20

Pumpkin Pie Soap

Materials

- 10 oz. olive oil

- 20 oz. coconut oil

- 8 oz. distilled water

- 4.73 oz. pure lye

- 3 oz. pure pumpkin puree

- 3 tablespoons pumpkin pie spice– this is optional, but if you omit it, your soap won't have much scent

- 15 drops clove essential oil

- 15 drops cinnamon OR cassia essential oil (optional)

- Safety gear for handling lye (long-sleeve shirt, gloves, safety glasses, etc.)

- Equipment for making hot process soap

Directions

Follow your favorite hot process soap making recipe such as the one found here: http://www.theprairiehomestead.com/2015/10/pumpkin-soap-recipe.html

October 21

Aromatic Fall Scented Sachet

Materials

- Small sachet sack
- Thin ribbon or raffia
- ½ cup uncooked rice
- Favorite fall perfume

Directions

Add the rice to a bowl followed by a few splashes of your favorite woodsy or spicy perfume. Mix the rice and perfume together. Pour the mixture into the sachet and secure with the ribbon or raffia. Place in linen closets or drawers.

October 22

Apple Pie Diffuser Blend

Materials

- 2 drops clove bud
- 2 drops cinnamon bark
- 2 drops ginger

Directions

Add all essential oil to your diffuser.

October 23

Fall Retreat Diffuser Blend

Materials

- 3 drops orange
- 2 drops frankincense
- 2 drops cassia

Directions

Add all essential oil to your diffuser.

October 24

Crisp, Fall Day Cuddles Diffuser Blend

Materials

- 3 drops cinnamon bark
- 2 drops clove bud
- 2 drops white fir

Directions

Add all essential oil to your diffuser.

October 25

Spiced Cider Diffuser Blend

Materials

- 4 drops orange

- 3 drops ginger

- 3 drops cinnamon

Directions

Add all essential oil to your diffuser.

October 26

Fall Flannel Shirt Diffuser Blend

Materials

- 5 drops bergamot

- 3 drops orange

- 3 drops Stress Away Blend by Young Living Oils

Directions

Add all essential oil to your diffuser.

October 27

Snickerdoodle Diffuser Blend

Materials

- 5 drops orange

- 2 drops cinnamon

- 1 drop clove

Directions

Add all essential oil to your diffuser.

October 28

Mulled Cider Diffuser Blend

Materials

- 4 drops orange
- 2 drops nutmeg
- 1 drop cinnamon bark
- 1 drop clove

Directions

Add all essential oil to your diffuser.

October 29

Sweater Weather Diffuser Blend

Materials

- 5 drops orange
- 4 drops Thieves blend by Young Living Oils
- 1 drop ginger

Directions

Add all essential oil to your diffuser.

October 30

Candy Bowl Diffuser Blend

Materials

- 6 drops cinnamon bark
- 3 drops tangerine

Directions

Add all essential oil to your diffuser.

October 31

Trick or Treat Diffuser Blend

Materials

- 3 drops orange
- 2 drops clove
- 2 drops ginger
- 2 drops frankincense

Directions

Add all essential oil to your diffuser.

November

October has come and gone and with our bellies full of Halloween candy we jump right into the month of November. Soon, Thanksgiving Day will be upon us and along with it comes the scents of the season like sage, oregano, nutmeg, pine, and chestnuts. During this month we will focus on scents that make us feel thankful as well as continuing on our journey of Autumn aromas.

November 1

Fresh Stuffing Diffuser Blend

Materials

- 3 drops orange
- 2 drops sage
- 2 drops patchouli

Directions

Add all essential oil to your diffuser.

November 2

Mother's November Brew Diffuser Blend

Materials

- 2 drops pine
- 1 drop frankincense
- 1 drop patchouli
- 1 drop lavender

Directions

Add all essential oil to your diffuser.

November 3

Be Thankful, Dear Child Diffuser Blend

Materials

- 1 drop lavender
- 2 drops marjoram
- 1 drop orange
- 1 drop juniper

Directions

Add all essential oil to your diffuser.

November 4

Sweet, November Nights Diffuser Blend

Materials

- 3 drops orange
- 2 drops clove
- 1 drop cassia
- 1 drop ginger

Directions

Add all essential oil to your diffuser.

November 5

Pumpkin Bread Diffuser Blend

Materials

- 4 drops cardamom
- 2 drops cinnamon bark
- 1 drop cassia
- 1 drop wild orange
- 1 drop clove

Directions

Add all essential oil to your diffuser.

November 6

Spiced Tea Diffuser Blend

Materials

- 4 drops orange
- 3 drops lemon
- 3 drops ginger
- 3 drops cinnamon
- 1 drop tea tree

Directions

Add all essential oil to your diffuser.

November 7

Harvest Time Diffuser Blend

Materials

- 6 drops orange
- 2 drops ginger
- 1 drop patchouli
- 1 drop sage

Directions

Add all essential oil to your diffuser.

November 8

Turkey Dinner Diffuser Blend

Materials

- 1 drop black pepper
- 1 drop lemon
- 1 drop basil
- 1 drop orange
- 1 drop clove

Directions

Add all essential oil to your diffuser.

November 9

Run into The Woods Diffuser Blend

Materials

- 1 drop arborvitae

- 1 drop cedarwood

- 2 drops frankincense

Directions

Add all essential oil to your diffuser.

November 10

Fresh, Baked Pumpkin Pie Recipe

Materials

- ¾ cup sugar

- 1 ½ tsp. pumpkin pie spice

- ½ tsp. salt

- 1 can pumpkin puree

- 1 ¼ cups evaporated milk

- 2 eggs, beaten

- 1 frozen deep-dish crust

Directions

Heat your oven to 435 degrees. In a large bowl, mix the filling ingredients and pour into frozen pie crust. Bake pie for 15 minutes, and then reduce temperature to 350 degrees. Continue baking for 40 to 50 minutes or until a knife or toothpick comes out clean when inserted into the middle. Nothing beats the smell of a pumpkin pie cooling on the counter on a crisp, fall day.

November 11

November Day Diffuser Blend

Materials

- 4 drops On-Guard blend by DoTerra Oils
- 2 drops cloves
- 2 drops juniper berry
- 2 drops wild orange

Directions

Add all essential oil to your diffuser.

November 12

Peaceful, November Night's Sleep Diffuser Blend

Materials

- 3 drops vetiver
- 3 drops Serenity Blend by DoTerra Oils

Directions

Add all essential oil to your diffuser.

November 13

Vivid Dreams Diffuser Blend

Materials

- 5 drops clary sage
- 5 drops patchouli

Directions

Add all essential oil to your diffuser.

November 14

No More Grouchies Diffuser Blend

Materials

- 3 drops Balance blend by DoTerra
- 3 drops lavender

Directions

Add all essential oil to your diffuser.

November 15

Autumn Zing Diffuser Blend

Materials

- 3 drops cardamom
- 2 drops orange
- 1 drop cinnamon

- 1 drop clove
- 1 drop wintergreen

Directions

Add all essential oil to your diffuser.

November 16

Thanksgiving Dinner Diffuser Blend

Materials

- 3 drops Holiday Joy Blend by DoTerra Oils
- 2 drops clove
- 1 drop lemon

Directions

Add all essential oil to your diffuser.

November 17

Oatmeal Cookie Diffuser Blend

Materials

- 3 drops orange
- 2 drops cassia
- 2 drops cedarwood

Directions

Add all essential oil to your diffuser.

November 18

Give Thanks Diffuser Blend

Materials

- 4 drops cypress

- 2 drops white fir

- 2 drops sandalwood

Directions

Add all essential oil to your diffuser.

November 19

Orange Pomander Diffuser Blend

Materials

- 3 drops orange

- 2 drops clove

- 2 drops rosemary

Directions

Add all essential oil to your diffuser.

November 20

Thankful Heart Diffuser Blend

Materials

- 1 drop ginger
- 1 drop cinnamon bark
- 2 drops coriander
- 1 drop clove

Directions

Add all essential oil to your diffuser.

November 21

Orange Glow Diffuser Blend

Materials

- 4 drops orange
- 1 drop cassia

Directions

Add all essential oil to your diffuser.

November 22

Fresh, Fall Home Diffuser Blend

Materials

- 3 drops basil

- 2 drops cinnamon bark

- 2 drops lime

Directions

Add all essential oil to your diffuser.

November 23

Here Comes the Harvest Sun Diffuser Blend

Materials

- 1 drop sage

- 3 drops bergamot

- 2 drops orange

- 2 drops ginger

Directions

Add all essential oil to your diffuser.

November 24

Northern Lights Diffuser Blend

Materials

- 2 drops juniper berry

- 2 drops lemongrass

- 4 drops wintergreen

Directions

Add all essential oil to your diffuser.

November 25

Under the Blankets Diffuser Blend

Materials

- 3 drops cinnamon leaf
- 2 drops orange
- 1 drop clove
- 1 drop nutmeg
- 1 drop vanilla

Directions

Add all essential oil to your diffuser.

November 26

Pumpkin Latte Diffuser Blend

Materials

- 4 drops cardamom
- 2 drops wild orange
- 1 drop cinnamon
- 1 drop clove
- 1 drop ginger

Directions

Add all essential oil to your diffuser.

November 27

Fall Festival Diffuser Blend

Materials

- 6 drops patchouli
- 4 drops orange
- 2 drops lavender

Directions

Add all essential oil to your diffuser.

November 28

Pumpkin Spice Pot Simmer

Materials

- 20 drops cinnamon
- 15 drops nutmeg
- 15 drops ginger
- 15 drops clove
- 10 drops orange
- 5 drops cardamom
- 3 small pine cones
- 1 large sprig of rosemary

- 4 cups water

Directions

Add all ingredients to a medium-sized pot on the stove and heat over medium-low heat. Allow to simmer for at least 30 minutes.

November 29

Fall Travels Diffuser Blend

Materials

- 2 drops peppermint

- 2 drops wild orange

- 1 drop frankincense

Directions

Add all essential oil to your diffuser.

November 30

Cinnamon Creamsicle Diffuser Blend

Materials

- 4 drops sweet orange

- 3 drops cinnamon

- 2 drops vanilla

Directions

Add all essential oil to your diffuser.

December

Winter is here once again but never fear, Christmas in near! The month of December is all about having a joyful spirit in celebration of the holiday season. Warm, cozy, winter blends are some of the best aromatherapy experiences of the year. Grab your diffuser, fill it with one of these amazing blends, grab a book, and get cozy by the frosted window pain.

December 1

Christmas Tree Farm Diffuser Blend

Materials

- 3 drops douglas fir
- 2 drops cedarwood
- 1 drop juniper berry

Directions

Add all essential oil to your diffuser.

December 2

Christmas Candy Diffuser Blend

Materials

- 3 drops peppermint
- 2 drops wild orange
- 2 drops cassia
- 3 drops wintergreen

Directions

Add all essential oil to your diffuser.

December 3

Peaceful Holiday Farm Diffuser Blend

Materials

- 5 drops balsam fir
- 5 drops black spruce
- 2 drops cedarwood
- 1 drop juniper berry

Directions

Add all essential oil to your diffuser.

December 4

Spicy Christmas Candy Diffuser Blend

Materials

- 2 drops wintergreen
- 2 drops peppermint
- 2 drops cinnamon
- 1 drop orange

Directions

Add all essential oil to your diffuser.

December 5

Winter Christmas Tree Diffuser Blend

Materials

- 3 drops blue spruce
- 4 drops cedarwood
- 4 drops pine

Directions

Add all essential oil to your diffuser.

December 6

Winter Wonder Diffuser Blend

Materials

- 5 drops orange
- 5 drops spruce
- 3 drops pine

Directions

Add all essential oil to your diffuser.

December 7

Solstice Celebration Diffuser Blend

Materials

- 4 drops pine

- 3 drops frankincense
- 2 drops orange
- 2 drops juniper
- 2 drops cypress
- 1 drop clove

Directions

Add all essential oil to your diffuser.

December 8

Winter Happiness Diffuser Blend

Materials

- 10 drops orange
- 5 drops cedarwood
- 1 drop ylang ylang

Directions

Add all essential oil to your diffuser.

December 9

Orange Cream Diffuser Blend

Materials

- 4 drops orange
- 2 drops cedarwood

Directions

Add all essential oil to your diffuser.

December 10

Candy Cane Diffuser Blend

Materials

- 4 drops peppermint
- 2 drops spearmint

Directions

Add all essential oil to your diffuser.

December 11

Black Licorice Diffuser Blend

Materials

- 4 drops fennel
- 2 drops Pan Away Blend by Young Living Oils

Directions

Add all essential oil to your diffuser.

December 12

Gingerbread Man Diffuser Blend

Materials

- 4 drops cardamom
- 2 drops Christmas Spirit Blend by Young Living Oils

Directions

Add all essential oil to your diffuser.

December 13

Santa's Workshop Diffuser Blend

Materials

- 3 drops sweet orange
- 2 drops peppermint
- 2 drops fir needle
- 1 drop cinnamon leaf
- 1 drop clove bud

Directions

Add all essential oil to your diffuser.

December 14

Candy Cane Forest Diffuser Blend

Materials

- 3 drops fir needle

- 2 drops peppermint

- 2 drops orange

- 1 drop wintergreen

- 1 drop cedarwood

Directions

Add all essential oil to your diffuser.

December 15

Sea of Swirly Twirly Gumdrops Diffuser Blend

Materials

- 2 drops lemon

- 2 drops tangerine

- 1 drop cinnamon leaf

- 1 drop clove bud

- 1 drop spearmint

- 1 drop aniseed

Directions

Add all essential oil to your diffuser.

December 16

Christmas Coffee Diffuser Blend

Materials

- 4 drops coffee oil
- 1 drop patchouli
- 1 drop cardamom
- 1 drop nutmeg

Directions

Add all essential oil to your diffuser.

December 17

Snow Angels Diffuser Blend

Materials

- 2 drops peppermint
- 2 drops juniper berry
- 1 drop wintergreen
- 1 drop fir needle
- 1 drop eucalyptus

Directions

Add all essential oil to your diffuser.

December 18

Christmas Cheer Diffuser Blend

Materials

- 2 drops for needle
- 2 drops frankincense
- 2 drops tangerine
- 2 drops cinnamon leaf

Directions

Add all essential oil to your diffuser.

December 19

Christmas Cookie Recipe

Materials

- 1 ½ cups butter, softened
- 2 cups white sugar
- 4 eggs
- 1 tsp. vanilla extract
- 5 cups all-purpose flour
- 2 tsps. baking powder
- 1 tsp. salt

Directions

In a large bowl, cream together butter and sugar until smooth. Then, beat in the eggs and vanilla. Stir in the flour, baking powder, and salt. Cover, and chill dough for at least 1 hour or even overnight.

Preheat oven to 400 degrees. Roll out dough on a floured surface about ½ inch thick. Cut into shapes using Christmas cookie cutters. Place onto ungreased baking sheets and bake for 6-8 minutes. Allow to completely cool before decorating.

Enjoy the aromatic scent of freshly baked cookies wafting through your home.

December 20

Peppermint Surprise Diffuser Blend

Materials

- 2 drops peppermint
- 2 drops ylang ylang

Directions

Add all essential oil to your diffuser.

December 21

Cuddle by The Fire Diffuser Blend

Materials

- 2 drops white fir
- 2 drops cinnamon
- 1 drop clove
- 1 drop cedarwood

Directions

Add all essential oil to your diffuser.

December 22

All is Calm, All is Bright Diffuser Blend

Materials

- 3 drops Peace and Calming blend by Young Living Oils
- 3 drops peppermint

Directions

Add all essential oil to your diffuser.

December 23

Gifts of the Magi Diffuser Blend

Materials

- 2 drops frankincense
- 2 drops myrrh
- 2 drops wild orange

Directions

Add all essential oil to your diffuser.

December 24

Christmas Eve Diffuser Blend

Materials

- 5 drops pine
- 3 drops frankincense

- 3 drops sweet orange

- 3 drops peppermint

- 2 drops cinnamon

- 2 drops roman chamomile

- 1 drop clove

- 1 drop cedarwood

- Toothpick of birch tar – dip toothpick into essential oil and swirl into the blend.

Directions

Add all essential oil to your diffuser.

December 25

Christmas Day Diffuser Blend

Materials

- 3 drops white fir

- 2 drops grapefruit

- 2 drops frankincense

Directions

Add all essential oil to your diffuser.

December 26

Calming Winter Diffuser Blend

Materials

- 3 drops wild orange
- 2 drops cedarwood
- 1 drop ylang ylang

Directions

Add all essential oil to your diffuser.

December 27

Winter Comfort Diffuser Blend

Materials

- 3 drops orange
- 2 drops cassia
- 2 drops cedarwood

Directions

Add all essential oil to your diffuser.

December 28

Blessings Diffuser Blend

Materials

- 2 drops sweet orange
- 2 drops cedarwood

- 1 drop frankincense
- 1 drop myrrh

Directions

Add all essential oil to your diffuser.

December 29

Nutcracker Diffuser Blend

Materials

- 3 drops tangerine
- 3 drops white fir

Directions

Add all essential oil to your diffuser.

December 30

Frosty Morning Diffuser Blend

Materials

- 3 drops peppermint
- 3 drops wild orange

Directions

Add all essential oil to your diffuser.

December 31

Happy New Year Diffuser Blend

Materials

- 3 drops bergamot
- 1 drop ylang ylang
- 1 drop grapefruit

Directions

Add all essential oil to your diffuser.

<u>Conclusion</u>

We hope you have enjoyed this wonderful book filled with aromatherapy recipes. When you incorporate the gift of aromatherapy into your daily life, you'll begin see many positive changes taking place. What we smell plays a big part in how we feel. Give yourself a great start to each day by using a special diffuser blend to invigorate your senses.

Remember, aromatherapy doesn't only manifest through your diffuser. You can create homemade massage oils, bath oils, body balms, and cleaning products using your favorite essential oils. Give yourself a dose of aromatherapy as you go about your day-to-day duties.

As always, if you should notice any adverse effects from using a particular aromatherapy blend, immediately discontinue use and consult your health care provider. Always use caution when using aromatherapy in children, the elderly, and pregnant mothers.